ABC OF UROLOGY

Second Edition

ABC OF UROLOGY

Second Edition

Edited by

Chris Dawson
Consultant Urological Surgeon, Edith Cavell Hospital, Peterborough

Hugh N Whitfield
Consultant Urological Surgeon, Harold Hopkins Department of Urology, Royal Berkshire Hospital, Reading

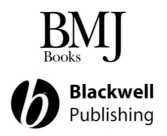

BMJ Books

Blackwell Publishing

© Blackwell Publishing Ltd 2006
BMJ Books is an imprint of the BMJ Publishing Group, used under licence

Blackwell Publishing Inc., 350 Main Street, Malden, Massachusetts 02148–5020, USA
Blackwell Publishing Ltd, 9600 Garsington Road, Oxford OX4 2DQ, UK
Blackwell Publishing Asia Pty Ltd, 550 Swanston Street, Carlton, Victoria 3053, Australia

First published 1997
Second edition 2006

2   2008

Library of Congress Cataloging-in-Publication Data
ABC of urology / edited by Chris Dawson, Hugh N. Whitfield. — 2nd ed.
        p. ; cm.
     "BMJ Books."
     Includes bibliographical references and index.
     ISBN: 978-1-4051-3959-5
   1. Urology. 2. Genitourinary organs — Diseases. I. Dawson, Chris, MBBS.
II. Whitfield, Hugh N.
        [DNLM: 1. Urologic Diseases — diagnosis. 2. Urologic
Diseases — therapy. 3. Genital Diseases, Male — diagnosis. 4. Genital
Diseases, Male — WJ 140 A134 2006]

     RC871.A13 2006
     616.6—dc22

                              2006012216

A catalogue record for this book is available from the British Library

Cover image of a urinary tract x-ray is courtesy of Sovereign, ISM/Science Photo Library

Set in 9/11 pts New Baskerville by Newgen Imaging System Pvt., Ltd, Chennai, India
Printed and bound in Singapore by C.O.S. Printers Pte Ltd

Commissioning Editor: Eleanor Lines
Editorial Assistant: Vicky Pittman
Development Editor: Sally Carter / Vicki Donald
Production Controller: Debbie Wyer

For further information on Blackwell Publishing, visit our website:
www.blackwellpublishing.com

Contents

Contributors   vi

Preface   vii

Introduction to urology   ix

1   Urological evaluation   1
Hugh N Whitfield

2   Bladder outflow obstruction   6
Jyoti Shah

3   Urinary incontinence   10
Helen Zafirakis-Hegarty

4   Urological emergencies   14
Adam Jones

5   Subfertility and male sexual dysfunction   18
Stephanie Symons

6   Management of urinary tract infection in adults   22
Philippa Cheetham

7   Prostate cancer   25
Chris Dawson

8   Bladder cancer   29
Derek Fawcett

9   Renal and testis cancer   34
Paul K Hegarty

10   Urinary tract stone disease   37
Hugh N Whitfield

11   Common paediatric problems   40
A R Prem

12   Genitourinary trauma   44
Asif Muneer

Index   49

Contributors

Philippa Cheetham
Specialist Registrar in Urology, Harold Hopkins Department of Urology, Royal Berkshire Hospital, Reading

Chris Dawson
Consultant Urological Surgeon, Edith Cavell Hospital, Peterborough

Derek Fawcett
Consultant Urological Surgeon, Harold Hopkins Department of Urology, Royal Berkshire Hospital, Reading

Paul K Hegarty
Specialist Registrar Urology, Great Ormond Street Hospital, London

Adam Jones
Consultant Urological Surgeon, Harold Hopkins Department of Urology, Royal Berkshire Hospital, Reading

Asif Muneer
Specialist Registrar in Urology, Harold Hopkins Department of Urology, Royal Berkshire Hospital, Reading

A R Prem
Senior Registrar in Urology, The Armed Forces Hospital, Al-Khoud, Sultanate of Oman

Jyoti Shah
Specialist Registrar in Urology, Northwick Park Hospital, Harrow

Stephanie Symons
Specialist Registrar in Urology, Edith Cavell Hospital, Peterborough

Hugh N Whitfield
Consultant Urological Surgeon, Harold Hopkins Department of Urology, Royal Berkshire Hospital, Reading

Helen Zafirakis-Hegarty
Specialist Registrar in Urology, Edith Cavell Hospital, Peterborough

Preface

There have been considerable technical and scientific innovations since the publication of the first edition of the *ABC of Urology* nearly 10 years ago. The time is therefore right for the publication of this revised second edition.

Acknowledging the progress made in each area of urology we felt that it was appropriate for us to take on an editorial role and invite specialist authors each to contribute to their area of expertise. Each chapter has been completely rewritten and contains up to date information contributed by an expert in the field. We hope that this edition will be the more authoritative as a result.

The *ABC of Urology* remains a useful introduction to the subject for surgeons training for the MRCS and will also provide a source of information for medical students. The style of each chapter also means that this book will prove a useful resource for nursing and ancillary staff dealing with patients with urological problems.

We remain indebted to the staff of Blackwell Publishing without whose efforts this revised edition would not have been possible.

Chris Dawson and Hugh N Whitfield

Introduction to urology

Hugh N Whitfield

Urological disorders account for about one third of all surgical admissions to hospital. Urological pathology is also a common reason for patients to present in primary care. Although few urological conditions are immediately life threatening, many may have a profound effect on the patient's quality of life.

As with all other medical and surgical specialties, subspecialisation has occurred within urological practice. Evidence in the confidential enquiry into perioperative deaths (CEPOD) highlighted that transurethral prostatectomy, the operation performed most often in urological departments, is associated with a significantly lower mortality when performed by surgeons who undertake more than 50 such procedures a year. Most urologists will undertake core urology and will subspecialise in one or two of the component parts of urology. One common theme is that urological surgery requires specialised urological nursing to be effective

Urodynamic disorders

Problems of bladder outflow obstruction secondary to benign prostatic hypertrophy constitute about one third of cases in urological practice. Other urodynamic disorders occur in patients with neurological disorders of many kinds. The management of patients with urinary incontinence may also be included under this heading, although urogynaecologists are now taking over a considerable part of this workload.

Oncology

Prostate and bladder cancer are the two most common malignant diseases that present to urologists. The numbers of renal and testicular cancers that are being found seems to be increasing. All patients with malignant diseases now come under the care of a multidisciplinary team that consists of urologists, oncologists, radiologists, and histopathologists. Urological oncologist nurses have an increasing role to play in the counselling and follow-up of patients with malignant disease.

Stone disease

In most urological departments with five or more urologists, one urologist will have a subspecialty interest in stone disease. The need for expensive technology dictates that the most comprehensive care for patients with stone disease can be provided only in centres with an onsite lithotripter and equipment for endoscopic treatments, including lasers. Such a capital investment can be justified only for a population base of 750 000–1 000 000.

Reconstruction

Paediatric urologists are responsible for managing congenital anomalies that need urological reconstruction. In adult practice, urethral stricture disease remains a challenge. After radical cystectomy for bladder cancer, some patients with incontinence can be offered a reconstructive procedure that may be performed by an oncological or reconstructive surgeon. A few

Subspecialties in urology
- Urodynamics
- Oncology
- Stone disease
- Reconstruction
- Paediatric urology
- Andrology

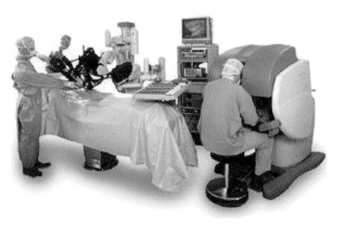

A robotic laparoscopy system

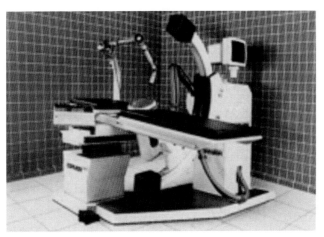

A lithotripter

patients with intractable urological incontinence may also be offered a reconstructive procedure. Uncommon problems involving the ureters also may require a reconstructive procedure, with the small intestine used to substitute for the ureter.

Paediatric urology

Paediatric urological disorders are managed best by those with special expertise in the investigation, surgery, and nursing of children. The regulations that surround the care of children are creating a situation in which it is increasingly difficult for an adult urologist to undertake any paediatric urology. This is not always appropriate, as the small number of paediatric urologists, at least in the United Kingdom, should be devoting their time to problems more complex than phimosis and undescended testicle, which can be managed very well by non-specialists.

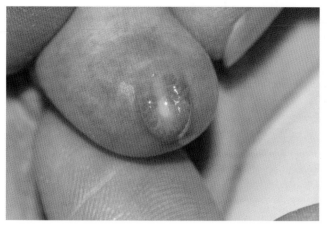

Balanitis and phimosis in a 5 year old boy. Reproduced with permission from Dr P Marazzi/Science Photo Library

Andrology

The role of the urologist in the management of erectile dysfunction and subfertility is changing. With the advent of oral agents to treat most patients with erectile dysfunction, much of this component of urology has been taken on by primary care doctors. Urologists who subspecialise in andrology may be more involved in the surgery of patients with severe Peyronie's disease and those who request gender reassignment.

Renal transplantation

In most centres, dedicated transplant surgeons are responsible for renal transplantation. Urologists become involved only in cases in which patients have postoperative ureteric problems or renal stone disease.

Changes in urological practice

In the last 10 years many changes have resulted in a considerable shift in the scope of urological care. More effective medical treatment for benign prostatic hyperplasia has resulted in a reduction in the number of operations required for this common problem. As mentioned above, specialists from other disciplines are playing an increasing role in the management of andrological disorders and of urodynamic disorders in women.

Laparoscopic surgery is performed increasingly within urology. The dilemma arises to decide whether laparoscopic surgeons will remain organ and pathology based or technique based.

As the requirement for urological specialists to perform surgery is diminishing, the training of urologists must adapt to accommodate these changes. Just starting in the United Kingdom is a two stage system; a three year training in core urology to produce a "consultant urologist" will start after basic surgical training. The scope of the surgery that consultant urologists undertake will be limited. Those who wish to become urological surgeons will have to hope that manpower calculations show a need before they undertake a further period of training for two or three years in a urological surgical subspecialty. Currently, the United Kingdom has a lower ratio of urologists per head of the population than any other developed country.

Male factor infertility

- Some centres have a combined clinic, in which a gynaecologist and urologist see both partners at the same time
- Gynaecologists are now undertaking much of the care of men with subfertility, although surgery for vasal blockage and varicocoele remain the remit of urologists

---

Ratio of urologists to population

Country	Ratio
Luxembourg	1:27 000
United States	1:29 000
Czech Republic	1:29 000
Spain	1:35 000
Portugal	1:40 000
Belgium	1:40 000
Netherlands	1:56 000
United Kingdom	1:100 000

Philosophy of urology

The investigation and treatment of patients with urological disorders tends to be minimally invasive. The urological equivalent of diagnostic laparotomy seldom, if ever, is needed. Most of even the most major urological surgical procedures may be performed laparoscopically. This will become the standard in the next few years.

The pharmaceutical industry is anticipating an increase in the proportion of medically treated urological disorders: from 5% to 15% over the next 10 years. With an ageing population and increased expectation for quality of life, the demand for medical and surgical urological care is likely to increase. Manpower predictions for training purposes will become increasingly complex.

Shared care between urologists and primary care doctors is common and effective. Integration with other healthcare professionals—such as district nurses, physiotherapists, radiographers, and urology nurse practitioners based in hospitals—also has a pivotal role. One recent example of close collaboration is the setting up of multidisciplinary tumour group meetings to manage patients with urological cancers.

The provision of urological health is likely to shift in the next few years. The role of the "independent sector" in the provision of non-oncological urology is unclear, and the latter may become the "Cinderella" of the specialty.

Urologists have a reputation for innovation. Although innovations can be of great benefit to patients—for example, extracorporeal shock wave lithotripsy—the recent history of urology is littered with examples of technologies that have been introduced with great enthusiasm by their protagonists but abandoned after a short time. The advent of a scrutinising committee from the National Institute for Clinical Excellence should act to hold back those who are overenthusiastic.

Participants in shared care
- Urological surgeon
- General practitioner
- District nurses
- Continence nurses
- Stoma therapists

Participants in multidisciplinary teams
- Urological surgeons
- Oncologists
- Radiotherapists
- Histopathologists
- Radiologists
- Nurse oncologists

Urological provision is changing
- More care based in community
- Emergency care provided by emergency departments of district general hospitals
- Elective surgery for oncology available at centres that provide care for populations of about 1 million people

1 Urological evaluation

Hugh N Whitfield

Urological complaints

The most common urological complaints that trigger the need for referral to a primary care doctor or urological surgeon can be divided into those referable to the lower urinary tract and those referable to the upper urinary tract. Although a careful history may be diagnostic in patients with, for example, renal colic or testicular torsion, very often non-specific features are more difficult to unravel.

Symptoms

The bladder has been described as an unreliable witness. Sensory innervation is mediated largely through parasymapathetic nerves, with pain from overdistension mediated through the sympathetic nervous system. The precision with which the site and cause of symptoms in the lower and upper urinary tracts can be identified from this autonomic innervation is limited. Similar symptoms may occur as the result of different pathology. The art of urological evaluation on the basis of symptoms depends on understanding how much reliance can be placed on the patient's account of different symptoms and symptom complexes. This also depends on the ability of the doctor to phrase questions so that the patient is clear about their meaning.

Obstructive symptoms
Hesitancy of micturition can be a reliable symptom. The patient can quantify accurately a delay in initiation of the urinary stream. Using quite crude analogies, most men can describe whether their urinary stream is fast or slow—that is, strong or weak. A man's ability to write his initials with his urine on the wall behind a urinal indicates a strong stream, whereas a stream that dribbles onto his toes obviously is weak. Patients can confirm if their urinary stream is intermittent, and this is a good indicator of obstruction. A feeling of incomplete bladder emptying correlates poorly with objective findings on ultrasound.

Irritative symptoms
A burning sensation on micturition is common in patients with a lower urinary tract infection. A similar sensation can occur in the absence of infection, however, and infection can occur in the absence of any discomfort.

The term "dysuria" is often applied to a burning sensation on micturition, but it means different things to different people and is best avoided. Urgency of micturition may be sensory or motor in origin, but when a history is taken, it is hard to distinguish between the two—although the underlying pathologies are very different. Patients with urgency feel as if they may leak urine if they are not able to reach a lavatory imminently. The sensation of needing to pass urine again just after micturition—strangury— is the urological equivalent of tenesmus. In the urinary tract, the symptom is not diagnostic for any one pathology.

Frequency of micturition
When patients are asked to describe their urinary frequency, they have every opportunity for an unhelpful and lengthy reply. The number of times a patient wakes to pass urine at night is a value that most people can identify accurately. A single episode

---

Differentiation between urological and non-urological causes of non-specific symptoms can be made only after basic urological investigation

---

Urological symptoms
- Obstructive symptoms
- Irritative symptoms
- Erectile dysfunction and sexual problems
- Urinary incontinence
- Pain
- Renal colic
- Fever
- Haematuria

Obstructive symptoms
- Hesitancy
- Poor stream
- Intermittent stream
- Terminal dribbling

Irritative symptoms
- Burning on micturition
- Urgency
- Daytime frequency
- Nocturia
- Urge incontinence

Input/Output Chart

Name..

Date...

Input		Output	
Time	Volume and type of fluid	Time	Volume

Recording frequency of micturition on a "time and volume" chart can be useful

of nocturia is within normal limits. More than this number becomes increasingly important.

Daytime urinary frequency is subject to so many variables that it almost is unhelpful—except to know whether such frequency provokes an adverse effect on the patient's lifestyle.

Urinary incontinence
To establish the circumstances under which urine loss occurs is important. Neither men nor women are entirely continent. In men, a small urinary leakage at the end of the stream (also known as "post-micturition dribble") is so common that it does not constitute an abnormality. Many women—young and old—leak a little urine on coughing. The degree of a patient's fastidiousness will dictate their response to minor degrees of urinary loss of this kind.

The single most important question to follow a complaint of urinary incontinence is "What protection do you need to cope with the leakage?" If the loss of urine needs no more than a change of underwear, further investigation is unlikely to be worthwhile, but referral for consideration of pelvic floor exercises may be beneficial to the patient.

Renal and ureteric colic
The pain from a stone that is moving within the urinary tract is among the most severe pains that patients may experience. Stones may move within the renal collecting system, and, in such cases, the pain is likely to be felt mainly in the loin. When a stone moves into the ureter, the pain may radiate into the iliac fossa and the scrotum or labia. The site of the pain, however, is not a very reliable indicator of the site of the stone.

Fever
Lower urinary tract infections do not cause a fever, which occurs only when a urinary infection is in a solid organ (kidney, prostate, or testis) or if the patient has an obstructed and infected urinary tract. The latter is an emergency that needs immediate nephrostomy drainage (under local anaesthesia). If an infected and obstructed kidney is suspected, urgent ultrasound (to confirm hydronephrosis) should be followed by percutaneous nephrostomy.

Sexual dysfunction
Erectile dysfunction presents as an inability to initiate or sustain an erection sufficient to enable vaginal penetration and subsequent orgasm. The presence of nocturnal or early morning erections makes an organic cause of erectile dysfunction less likely.

Retrograde ejaculation occurs commonly in men after transurethral resection of the prostate and sometimes in those who have taken a adrenergic blockers. Failure of ejaculation may occur after sympathectomy or retroperitoneal surgery, as the sympathetic pathways to the prostate and seminal vesicles are interrupted. Premature ejaculation occurs most often as a functional problem.

Examination

Much of the genitourinary tract is hidden from view. This dictates that many decisions on management are usually possible only at a second outpatient visit, when the results of baseline investigations are available.

External genitalia
If a lax scrotum lies between the thighs, the scrotal contents can be delivered painlessly for examination by taking and

Urinary leakage
- Urinary leakage is more common in women than in men
- A severe degree of urge incontinence will probably cause a larger volume of urine loss than the most severe stress incontinence
- Some women are unable to identify how they leak
- Urinary leakage during sexual intercourse occurs in some women

When a stone enters the intramural ureter, patients often describe strangury, and, in men, discomfort may be felt at the tip of the penis

If a urinary tract infection is suspected the presence of nitrites and red cells on dipstick testing can be useful, although not unequivocal, confirmatory evidence

Ideally, antibiotics should not be prescribed until a urine culture has been taken

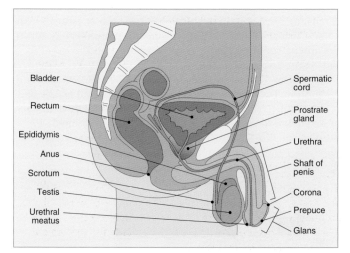

Male genitalia including scrotal contents. Reproduced from Adler M, et al. *ABC of sexually transmitted infections.* 5th edition. Oxford: Blackwell Publishing, 2004, and adapted from the *Sexually transmitted infections: history taking and examination* CD published by the Wellcome Trust, 2003.

pulling on a fold of scrotal skin. The testes appear without discomfort. The testes and epididymes can be identified separately.

If epididymal infection is present or testicular torsion is suspected, the examination must be extremely gentle to avoid causing pain. Observation of the colour of the scrotal wall may reveal hyperaemia. The absence of a cremasteric reflex contraction when the scrotum, or the area close to the scrotum, is touched is also an important sign to elicit. The loss of this reflex is not diagnostic of one pathology, but its presence is strongly against a diagnosis of torsion.

Examination of the penis should include assessment of the degree to which the prepuce can be retracted. The external urethral meatus must be identified: in patients with hypospadias and epispadias, the meatus will be sited abnormally. If an attempt is made to pull the sides of the meatus apart, the presence of meatal stenosis can be identified. The shaft of the penis is palpated to identify fibrous plaques of Peyronie's disease, which usually are found dorsally.

Rectal examination

To avoid causing the patient discomfort, rectal examination is performed best with the patient in the left lateral position. The examiner's finger should be inserted while the patient exhales to encourage maximum relaxation of the anal sphincter. The tone of the anal sphincter is noted, and in patients with incontinence as a result of weakness of the sphincter, it is helpful to ask the patient to contract their anal sphincter. Perianal sensation can be tested in the distribution of the S2, S3, and S4 segments—the spinal segments responsible for the main motor and sensory innervation of the bladder.

Examination of the prostate *per rectum* provides only a rough estimate of the size: the prostate can be categorised as small, medium, or large. The consistency of the prostate can be described as soft, firm, or hard; the surface as smooth or irregular; and the lateral lobes as symmetrical or asymmetrical. Although malignant prostates classically are hard, no precise correlation exists between any of the features described and a specific pathology. Although patients find examination of the prostate uncomfortable, only a bad examination technique, anal pathology, or inflamed prostate will cause significant discomfort or pain.

Initial investigations

Dipstick urine testing

Readily available and frequently used, dipstick testing of urine is a very inaccurate investigation. The presence of white cells and nitrites is only a rough guide to the presence of infection, although the absence of nitrites in the urine normally is enough to rule out an infection and the need for urine microscopy. Microscopic haematuria may be intermittent, but the presence of blood cells in the urine normally should prompt referral for further investigation, and it now is considered unnecessary to confirm the presence of red cells by urine microscopy.

Urine culture

Many laboratories now use an automated method to identify red and white cells in the urine. The numbers of each that can be considered normal are considerably higher than the numbers regarded as normal when urine microscopy is used. These values must be recognised, particularly for red cells, to prevent inappropriate referrals.

Urine cytology

Although some automation is used for the analysis of urine cytology, the final arbiter is microscopy—the accuracy of which

---

> The patient's external genitalia should be examined with the patient in the supine and erect positions to identify pathologies such as hernia and varicocele

---

Rectal examination

- Anal sphincter tone
- Anal sphincter contractility
- Peri-anal sensation
- Prostate—size, surface, symmetry, and consistency

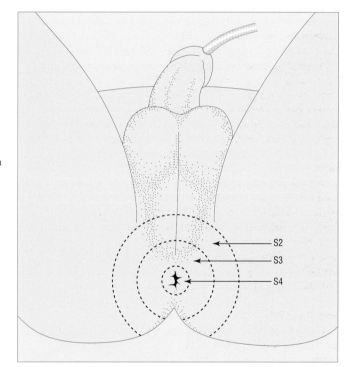

S2, S3, and S4 segments are responsible for the main motor and sensory innervation of the bladder

---

Initial investigations

- Urine culture
- Urine cytology
- Biochemistry
- Ultrasound
- Urodynamics
- Radiology
- Nuclear medicine

> Culture of a midstream specimen of urine is the only way to identify patients whose symptoms truly result from infection

depends on the expertise of the cytopathologist. Although alternatives to microscopy to identify malignant cells in urine have been introduced, none can reproduce the accuracy of the expert eye.

Biochemistry

Renal function is measured better by serum creatinine than by blood urea, the latter being influenced by the degree of hydration and rate of metabolism. The extent of reserve renal function means there must be a loss of two thirds of overall renal function before levels of serum creatinine increase. Measurements of sodium, potassium, and chloride electrolytes are the other baseline biochemical tests of relevance.

Ultrasound

Ultrasound examinations are used extensively now in the investigation of renal, ureteric, bladder, prostatic, and scrotal pathology. They may be regarded as an extension of examination. Whether an ultrasound examination is undertaken by an ultrasonographer, radiologist, or urologist, the person who undertakes the examination has the advantage of seeing the images in real time, while the doctor has only a few still images. The report thus is of prime importance, and the skill of the person who undertakes the examination is paramount. Limitations of ultrasound vary in different situations.

Kidney

In the kidney, ultrasound is better than computed tomography at identifying renal cysts, but it may fail to distinguish between parapelvic cysts and hydronephrosis. Although renal stones may give the classic appearance of a bright echo with a black shadow behind, this is not always the case. Ultrasound is a poor way of screening for renal stones. Assessment of the size of a stone using ultrasound is not very accurate. On occasions, if a stone fills the renal pelvis or the entire collecting system, it is possible to miss it on ultrasound. If the patient is obese, ultrasound becomes more difficult.

Bladder

The bladder is seen easily on transabdominal ultrasound, and volume measurements are easy and accurate. Intravesical pathology, such as tumours and stones, can be seen best when the bladder is full.

Prostate

Transrectal ultrasound of the prostate has transformed understanding of prostatic anatomy and pathology. Biopsies of the prostate and placement of radioactive seeds in brachytherapy are always undertaken with ultrasound imaging.

Scrotum

The scrotal contents are one of the few sites in urological practice where examination is easy. Differentiation between the normal epididymis and testis is accurate, and the vas can be palpated. In the presence of a tense hydrocele or inflammation, examination becomes more difficult and ultrasound may be worthwhile.

Ureter

Ureteric dilatation can be identified, but the cause is much more difficult to define. A stone at the lower end of the ureter may be identified by using the full bladder as an acoustic window.

Urological ultrasound
- Kidneys
- Ureters
- Bladder
- Prostate
- Scrotum

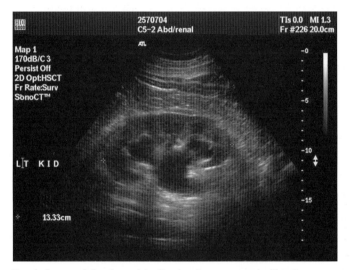

Renal ultrasound showing pelvi-caliceal and upper ureteric dilatation

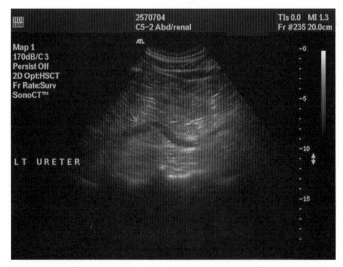

Ultrasound showing dilatated ureter

Urodynamics

Urodynamic investigations of the upper urinary tract are not commonly performed. Assessment of the function of the lower urinary tract can be made by a number of investigations:

- Urinary flow rate is a basic measurement that is obtained easily and non-invasively
- Assessment of bladder capacity and the size of the residual urine volume is made readily by cheap bladder scanners or more expensive ultrasound machines
- To add sophistication to a urodynamic assessment, bladder pressures can be measured with a urethral catheter during bladder filling and emptying
- Further information is afforded by performing a pressure or flow assessment under fluoroscopic imaging.

Radiological investigations

- Plain abdominal x ray
- Intravenous urogram
- Urethrogram
- Retrograde ureterogram
- Antegrade ureterogram
- Computed tomography
- Magnetic resonance imaging
- Isotope renogram
- Isotopic glomerular filtration rate
- Isotope bone scan

Radiological investigation

Intravenous urography

Intravenous urography (combined with renal ultrasound) remains the investigation of choice in patients with painless haematuria. New low osmolarity contrast media cause severe allergic reactions in less than 0.02% of patients.

Computed tomography

The use of computed tomography has increased in urological practice—often at the expense of increased doses of radiation. Computed tomography remains the investigation of choice for identification of renal masses. The rapid speed of the investigation offers advantages, but interpretation of images may need considerable investment of time at a sophisticated workstation that can format images in a wide variety of ways.

Magnetic resonance imaging

Magnetic resonance imaging has been adopted as the investigation of choice in the staging of prostate cancer. The same investigation can be helpful if used on bone settings to interpret areas of increased isotope uptake on a bone scan.

Positron emission tomography

Positron emission tomography is not available widely. It is not used routinely yet in urology.

Nuclear medicine

Dynamic isotope renography that uses mercaptoacetylglycine (MAG3) as the radiopharmaceutical is the most accurate method of identifying upper urinary tract obstruction and also shows differential renal function. Static renography with dimercaptosuccinic acid (DMSA) will identify renal scarring and differential renal function. The most accurate measurement of glomerular filtration rate is obtained by using an ethylenediaminetetraacetic acid (EDTA) clearance technique. Isotope bone scans are used in uro-oncology to identify bony metastatic disease.

> **Debate continues over whether intravenous urography is better than computed tomography for the investigation of patients with renal colic**

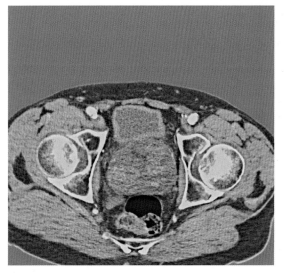

Axial coloured magnetic resonance image scan of a patient with prostate cancer. With permission from Du Cane Medical Imaging Ltd/ Science Photo Library

2 Bladder outflow obstruction

Jyoti Shah

Bladder outflow obstruction is most commonly the result of benign prostatic hyperplasia, which expands the transition zone of the prostate. This is part of the normal ageing process, and 10% of men in their 40s and up to 90% of men aged ≥ 80 years will have symptoms that are attributed to benign prostatic hyperplasia. Other causes of bladder outflow obstruction include urethral stricture, bladder neck obstruction, and bladder neck dyssynergia.

History

The assessment of a man with bladder outflow obstruction begins with a history. Traditionally, symptoms have been divided into irritative (related to storage of urine) and obstructive (voiding symptoms). The severity of symptoms can be quantified by the use of numerical symptoms scoring sheets such as the International prostate symptom score (IPSS).

Examination

All men should undergo a general physical examination that includes examination of the external genitalia. The cornerstone of the physical examination in patients with possible urological problems, however, is a digital rectal examination. This allows estimates of the size and consistency of the prostate gland.

Investigations

Urine should be sent for microscopy and culture to exclude a urinary tract infection. Haematuria should alert the doctor to other urological pathology that requires further evaluation. Serum electrolytes should also be requested. After discussion with the patient, an assay for prostate specific antigen should be requested, although this remains controversial.

Prostate specific antigen is a glycoprotein that is secreted by the epithelial cells that line the prostatic acini. Any disease process that interferes with the basement membrane of these cells will result in elevated levels of prostate specific antigen.

Symptoms of bladder outflow obstruction

Irritative symptoms	Obstructive symptoms
• Frequency	• Hesitancy
• Urgency	• Poor urine flow
• Nocturia	• Intermittent stream
• Incontinence	• Terminal dribbling
	• Incomplete emptying

Levels of prostate specific antigen adjusted for age

Age (years)	Normal range (ng/ml)
40–49	0–2.5
50–59	0–3.5
60–69	0–4.5
70–79	0–6.5

Alternative tests for prostate specific antigen

Test	Description
Free: total prostate specific antigen	• Prostate specific antigen exists in two forms in serum—free and bound to circulating proteins • A greater proportion of prostate specific antigen is protein-bound in patients with prostate cancer than in those with benign prostatic hyperplasia, which results in decreased free: total prostate specific antigen ratio • General cut off for prostate cancer is 0.15 (15%), below which the probability of cancer is high • Alternative assay for complexed prostate specific antigen measures the amount of prostate specific antigen that is protein bound
Prostate specific antigen density	• Density calculated by dividing level of prostate specific antigen by volume of prostate gland • Prostate biopsy advocated in patients with ratio >0.15
Prostate specific antigen velocity	• Refers to rate of change of prostate specific antigen over time • Patients with prostate cancer are thought to have more rapidly increasing levels of prostate specific antigen than those who do not have prostate cancer • An increase of >0.75 ng/ml a year suggests a higher risk of malignancy

International prostate symptom score

Questions				Score		
	Never	<1 time in 5	<50% of time	About 50% of time	More than 50% of time	Almost always
Symptoms of benign prostatic hyperplasia over past month						
Sensation that bladder is not empty after urinating	0	1	2	3	4	5
Need to urinate within two hours of previous urination	0	1	2	3	4	5
Need to stop and start again several times while urinating	0	1	2	3	4	5
Find it difficult to postpone urination	0	1	2	3	4	5
Have a weak urinary stream	0	1	2	3	4	5
Need to strain to urinate	0	1	2	3	4	5
Nocturia	**None**	**Once**	**Twice**	**3 times**	**4 times**	**≥5 times**
Number of times during night awakened by need to urinate	0	1	2	3	4	5

Scores are totalled: 7 or less = mild symptoms; 8 − 19 = moderate symptoms; 20 − 35 = severe symptoms.

The low specificity of assays for prostate specific antigen means that many researchers have developed alternative tests.

One of the most important investigations in patients suspected of having bladder outflow obstruction is measurement of the rate of urine flow and the volume of residual urine after the bladder is emptied. Normal bladder filling occurs up to a volume of 300–500 ml. The normal bladder, in the absence of outlet obstruction, empties to completion with a maximum flow rate of >15 ml/second. A poor flow rate is not proof of obstruction as a similar picture can be caused by detrusor failure.

A large residual volume (>300 ml) represents chronic retention of urine, with a risk of upper tract dilatation in cases of high pressure chronic retention. The kidneys of patients with residual volumes >200 ml should thus be evaluated by ultrasound investigation.

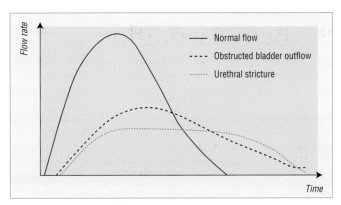

Typical traces produced in uroflowmetry in normal men, those with bladder outflow obstruction, and those with a stricture

Treatment

Watchful waiting
Not all patients with bladder outflow obstruction secondary to benign prostate hyperplasia need intervention. Their annual risk of developing acute urinary retention is 1–2%. As long as their symptoms are not bothersome and no complications of benign prostatic hyperplasia are present, observation is reasonable.

Pharmacological treatment
Plant extracts that contain saw palmetto are popular with men who have benign prostatic hyperplasia, although little evidence supports their use.

α Blockers such as tamsulosin, doxazosin, and alfuzosin relax prostatic smooth muscle and have a rapid onset of action. If they are going to produce a benefit, they will do so within four weeks of treatment being started. They can improve flow rates, although the improvement rarely is enough to restore the flow rate to the normal unobstructed range. The main side effect of α blockers is reductions in blood pressure, which can result in dizziness. They are therefore best taken before the patient goes to bed. Retrograde ejaculation can occur with α blockers. This is reversible when the drugs are stopped.

The 5α-reductase inhibitors (finasteride and dutasteride) must be taken for 3–6 months before they produce an effect. They are more effective in patients with large prostate glands (>50 g) and will reduce prostate volume by about 20%, thereby improving symptoms. The main side effects are loss of libido and erectile dysfunction, which occurs in 3% of patients.

Since the medical therapy of prostatic symptoms study (MTOPS) was undertaken, some evidence has shown that α blockers in combination with 5α-reductase inhibitors are more effective in managing symptoms than either treatment alone. Together, they also reduce the risk of acute urinary retention and the need for surgery for benign prostatic hyperplasia.

Surgical intervention
In the current climate, surgery is used for men who have failed medical pharmacological treatment or have had complications such as acute urinary retention.

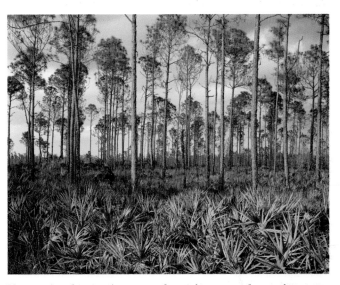

Plant extracts that contain extracts of saw palmetto are often used to treat benign prostatic hyperplasia. With permission from Jim Steinberg/Science Photo library

> "The evidence supporting combination therapy [for benign prostatic hyperplasia] in selected patients is so strong that I expect to see major changes in medical practice in the near future"
>
> **Leroy M Nyberg Jr**
> **Director of the urology program,**
> **National Institute of Diabetes and**
> **Digestive Kidney Diseases**
> **Adapted from NIH news release**
> **www.nih.gov/news/pr/may2002/niddk-28.htm**

Transurethral resection of prostate

This operation remains the gold standard for patients with benign prostatic hyperplasia. Most procedures involve a 1–2 day stay in hospital and provide improvement in symptom scores and flow rates. Although the complication rate is low, patients must be counselled adequately for this form of surgery.

Transurethral incision of prostate

Men with mild to moderate symptoms and a small prostate often have an elevated bladder neck. Such men will benefit from one or two incisions of the prostate from the ureteric orifices to the level of the verumontanum at the 5 o'clock and 7 o'clock positions. This operation is faster than transurethral resection of the prostate, and rates of retrograde ejaculation are lower (25%).

Laser therapy

The two main laser therapies use neodymium-doped yttrium aluminium garnet (Nd:Yag) and holmium-doped yttrium aluminium garnet (Holmium Yag) lasers. Both cause coagulative necrosis of the prostate tissue under direct vision with a cystoscope or ultrasound.

Photo selective vaporization of prostate with green light laser

Green light laser energy is absorbed by tissues and vessels rich in blood with only superficial penetration, which decreases postoperative irritative symptoms. The result is an almost bloodless operation that is performed as daycase surgery, with symptom improvement lasting up to five years. The mean time of catheterisation after the operation is 14 hours. At follow up at one year, the rate of retrograde ejaculation is 36% and the reoperation rate is 2.2%.

Transurethral microwave therapy

Microwave hyperthermia can be delivered to the prostate through transurethral catheters under local anaesthesia. Some reports have been made of improved symptom scores after transurethral microwave therapy, although the rate of postoperative urinary tract infections is high. This is possibly because patients are catheterised for longer after high-energy microwave therapy (average 1–2 weeks).

High intensity focused ultrasound

High intensity focused ultrasound is delivered through an ultrasound probe in the rectum. This heats the prostate and results in coagulative necrosis. This technique is less effective for bladder neck enlargement and median lobe enlargement and provides some improvement in symptom scores.

Transurethral needle ablation of the prostate

This technique uses interstitial radiofrequency to heat prostate tissue, which results in coagulative necrosis. As with high intensity focused ultrasound, transurethral needle ablation is ineffective for men who have large median lobes and high bladder necks. Some subjective and objective improvement occurs after transurethral needle ablation, although durability of the improvement is unknown.

Prostate stents

Intraurethral prostate stents that are placed with a flexible cystoscope under local anaesthetic are an excellent option for men who are elderly and need intervention but are high risk

Complications of transurethral resection of the prostate (TURP)

Complication	Rate (%)
Retrograde ejaculation	75
Erectile dysfunction	3–10
Incontinence	< 1
Transurethral resection syndrome	2
Repeat TURP needed	9

Laser therapy

Advantages

- Reduced blood loss
- Decreased incidence of transurethral resection syndrome
- Ability to perform the procedure as daycase surgery
- Reduced rate of retrograde ejaculation

Disadvantage

- Absence of tissue for pathological evaluation
- Long term results not known

Green light laser has a wavelength of 532 nm and is in the visible green part of spectrum

---

Cumulative reoperation rate after transurethral microwave therapy is 7%

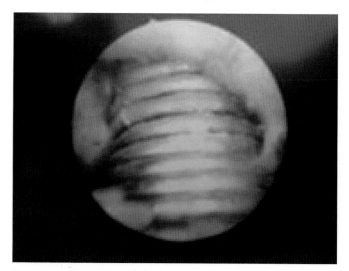
Prostate stent

candidates for anaesthesia. They are placed in the prostatic fossa but tend to be covered with urothelium within six months. They also can migrate and become heavily calcified.

Balloon dilatation
This technique uses a special catheter that results in dilatation of the prostatic fossa. The technique is used in men who have small prostates and provides relief of symptoms.

Open prostatectomy
This technique now is used only when the prostate is too large to be enucleated with endoscopic techniques. In general, prostate glands larger than 100 g are considered suitable for open prostatectomy.

Urethral stricture

Acquired urethral strictures are fibrotic narrowings of the urethra composed of collagen and fibroblasts. This restricts the flow of urine and may cause proximal urethral dilatation and bladder hypertrophy. A history of sexually transmitted diseases, urethral trauma, or previous catheterisation may be suggestive of urethral stricture. The trace produced by uroflowmetry in a patient with a urethral stricture is indicative of a stricture.

Treatment depends on the location, length, and degree of the urethral stricture. Options include dilatation, urethrotomy, or reconstruction for more complex or recurrent strictures.

Bladder neck dysfunction

Bladder outflow obstruction as a result of bladder neck dysfunction is also called bladder neck dyssynergia. This condition is almost exclusively found in young and middle aged men. Digital rectal examination tends to show a small and normal prostate gland. The condition is characterised by incomplete opening of the bladder neck during voiding, which produces an obstructed trace with urodynamics.

Medical treatment in the form of a blockers can relieve symptoms, although definitive treatment consists of bladder neck incision under cystoscopic vision. This carries a 15–50% risk of retrograde ejaculation, however, and requires careful consideration in young fertile men.

Summary

- Transurethral resection of prostate remains the gold standard treatment for bladder outflow obstruction as a result of benign prostatic hyperplasia
- Many minimally invasive techniques still need to be compared with transurethral resection of the prostate through randomised studies to provide data on durability, cost-effectiveness, and long term benefits

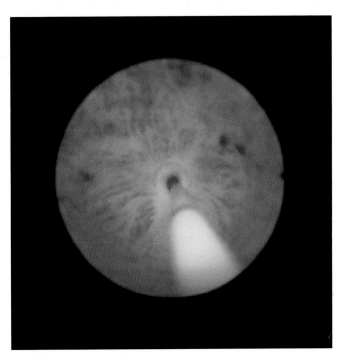

Endoscopic review of a tight bulbar urethral stricture, through which a guide wire is about to be passed before a urethrotomy

3 Urinary incontinence

Helen Zafirakis-Hegarty

Urinary incontinence is defined as the involuntary leakage of urine. The prevalence increases with age to about 14% in women and 13% in men aged 65–74 years. Various types of urinary incontinence exist.

Stress urinary incontinence is the involuntary leakage of urine from the urethra in association with exertion or effort, such as coughing and sneezing. Detrusor overactivity describes the involuntary contraction of the bladder and is usually associated with the symptom of urgency. Leakage of urine associated with this type of problem is known as urge incontinence. This generally is divided into neurogenic or non-neurogenic types. Patients with mixed incontinence often have features of stress and urge incontinence, usually with one type being predominant.

Overflow incontinence is caused by chronic retention of urine as a result of a non-painful bladder that is palpable on examination after voiding. Extraurethral incontinence implies leakage of urine through a fistula or an ectopic ureter. Patients typically void normally and are incontinent between voids (also known as paradoxical incontinence) The diagnosis and management of vesicovaginal fistula is covered in more detail at the end of this chapter.

Assessment

A detailed clinical history is of vital importance to establish the type of incontinence on the basis of symptoms and duration. The severity should be quantified in terms of the number of pads required by day and night. An assessment of quality of life will also determine the need for referral to a urologist. Inquiry into the past medical history should include questions related to frequency of urinary infections, parity, previous pelvic surgery, such as hysterectomy, and details of any drugs being taken.

Examination should include a physical examination as well as a neurological examination. The abdomen should be examined for a palpable bladder and scars from previous surgery. In women, examination of the perineum should look for atrophic vaginitis or signs of pelvic floor prolapse (such as cystocele, rectocele, vaginal vault, and uterine prolapse). Women should be asked to cough repeatedly with a full bladder to try to demonstrate stress urinary incontinence. An idea of pelvic floor strength can be gained by asking the patient to contract the pelvic floor while the examiner inserts two digits in the vagina—pelvic floor strength can be graded subjectively as weak, normal, or strong. In men, signs of phimosis or urethral meatal stenosis should be sought, and a digital rectal examination is mandatory to examine the prostate.

Urine analysis should be performed routinely in all patients. Further assessment can be performed by asking the patient to fill in a frequency or volume voided chart, which may be performed in primary care before referral. Other investigations include pad testing, uroflowmetry (with or without assessment of post micturition residual volume), and full urodynamics.

Causes of stress urinary incontinence

- Weakness of pelvic floor muscles (often as a result of childbirth)
- Intrinsic sphincter deficiency
- Damage of voluntary urethral sphincter (for example, after transurethral resection of prostate)
- Collagen disorders
- Advancing age

Neurogenic and non-neurogenic detrusor overactivity

Neurogenic causes	Non-neurogenic causes
• Spina bifida	• Thought to be the result of intrinsic problems within the bladder wall
• Multiple sclerosis	
• Spinal cord injury	
• Pelvic surgery	

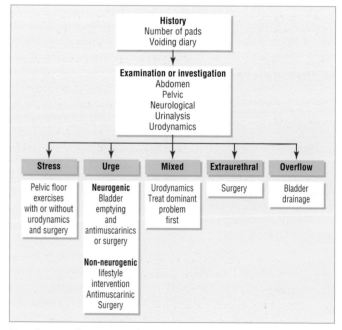

Flow diagram of assessment of incontinence

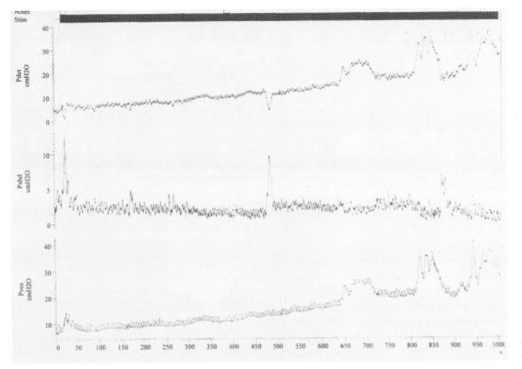

Typical recording from videourodynamic assessment

Urodynamic studies

Urodynamic studies examine the physiological behaviour of the bladder during filling and voiding. Small pressure transducing catheters are placed into the rectum and urethrally into the bladder. The bladder is filled with normal saline at body temperature.

Vesical pressure (P_{ves}) is calculated by subtracting the abdominal pressure (P_{abd}—actually the pressure measured by the probe in the rectum) from the detrusor pressure (P_{det}). During the filling phase, detrusor pressure is monitored to look for signs of detrusor overactivity. Stress incontinence can be provoked by asking the patient to cough during filling or by other provocative manoeuvres, include rapid filling and postural changes. The bladder capacity is recorded, and bladder compliance can also be determined from the change in detrusor pressure per unit volume.

During voiding, the detrusor pressure at maximum flow rate is recorded. The resulting flowmetry curve can also help in the diagnosis of obstruction.

Videourodynamics is similar to the above test, but it also uses contrast medium for bladder filling and can show anatomical abnormalities. This normally is reserved for patients with mixed incontinence or assessment of stress urinary incontinence before surgery.

Treatment

The treatment of incontinence ranges from non-surgical measures, such as pelvic floor training and biofeedback, to pharmacological methods, and surgery. Incontinence nurse practitioners are extremely useful allies in the non-surgical treatment of incontinence. Patients should also be made aware of support groups and organisations available for the various forms of incontinence.

Conservative treatment of stress incontinence

- Pelvic floor training can be easily taught to patients and is effective in up to 50% of patients
- It is normally taught by a physiotherapist or specialist nurse using vaginal cones of various sizes or biofeedback devices
- Exercises may need to be done regularly for a prolonged period if maximum benefit is to be obtained
- Devices that passively stimulate the pelvic floor are also available
- Other non-surgical treatments include urethral plugs, topical oestrogen replacement, or α agonists
- Duloxetine—a serotonin and noradrenaline reuptake inhibitor—was licensed for treatment of stress incontinence in September 2004 and can be used in primary care

---

Management of mixed urinary incontinence

- Clear understanding of main troublesome symptoms is vital, as is urodynamic assessment
- Conservative measures to control symptoms should be tried first
- Specialist care usually is preferable

Overflow incontinence

- Adequate bladder drainage is needed by:
  Intermittent self-catheterisation
  Long term catheterisation
  Bladder outflow surgery

Extraurethral incontinence

- Urinary fistulae need careful assessment followed by surgical repair

Usual practice is to treat the predominant symptoms first.

Surgical management of stress incontinence

A variety of surgical treatments exist for women with stress incontinence. The choice depends on the patient's age and parity, the degree of bladder neck mobility, previous surgery, and patient preference. Adequate preoperative assessment by a specialist is mandatory, and the patient must understand that more than one procedure may be needed.

In men with sphincter damage, pelvic floor exercises may have a role in the first instance, but the surgical treatment of choice is insertion of an artificial urethral sphincter. This involves placing an inflatable cuff around the urethra and a reservoir of fluid and a pump system normally in the scrotum. In its resting position, the cuff is inflated, which promotes continence. The patient activates the sphincter to allow the fluid to move back into the reservoir, which deflates the cuff and allows voiding to take place. The reservoir refills the cuff over a few minutes. This procedure should be performed only in specialist centres.

Management of detrusor instability

The mainstays of treatment for incontinence related to urge are bladder retraining and antimuscarinic drugs. Pelvic floor exercises may also be useful as part of bladder retraining, which involves teaching the patient to try to increase the time between voids. Antimuscarinic drugs inhibit the strength and frequency of unstable bladder contractions, thus reducing urgency and incontinence. They also allow the bladder to hold more volume. Treatment may be limited by side effects such as dry mouth and blurred vision. A number of such drugs are available, and the patient may have to try a number of these in sequence to provide the best results with the minimum of side effects.

Intractable urge incontinence may be treated with intravesical instillation of botulinum toxin, which is gaining in popularity. This treatment is not available in all centres, and the duration of effect is variable.

Surgical management for detrusor instability involves bladder augmentation with a piece of bowel (clam cystoplasty) or bladder myomectomy. These procedures often lead to incomplete bladder emptying and need intermittent self-catheterisation. As a result, these procedures are undertaken only after much consideration.

Vesicovaginal fistula

Vesicovaginal fistula is uncommon in the developed world. Most cases seen by urologists result from injury during gynaecological surgery. Three quarters of all such fistulae occur after abdominal or vaginal hysterectomy. Previous surgery to the uterus and a history of endometriosis or pelvic radiotherapy all are known to increase the risk of vesicovaginal fistula. In the developing world, vesicovaginal fistulae more commonly result from prolonged labour and trauma during childbirth.

Patients who develop vesicovaginal fistulae after pelvic surgery normally present with urinary leakage through the vagina within 7–10 days. In patients with more serious injury, immediate postoperative complications—such as paralytic ileus, flank tenderness, or haematuria—may develop. The latter symptoms are suggestive of ureteric obstruction or ureterovaginal fistula. Fistulae after pelvic radiotherapy may not develop for a number of years after the original insult.

Surgical management of stress incontinence in women

- Submucosal or periurethral injection treatment uses a bulking agent injected into the bladder neck or proximal urethra to increase urethral resistance. It is suitable only for patients with minimal bladder neck mobility; the effects are temporary in most cases
- Slings are very popular in patients with stress incontinence caused by intrinsic weakness of the sphincter, as well as those with considerable bladder neck mobility. Tension free vaginal tape especially is popular, with more than 700 000 cases having been performed with excellent results. Transobturator tapes also are available and are approved by the National Institute for Clinical Excellence. These can be done under general or local anaesthetic. Sling procedures can also employ donated or prepared tissue
- Birch colposuspension and vaginal obturator shelf procedure are open procedures with excellent long term results. They are the gold standard for patients with considerable mobility of the bladder neck. The procedure involves mobilisation of the vagina on either side of the bladder neck and suturing of the endopelvic fascia to the pectineal ligament or obturator fascia. This prevents descent of the bladder during straining

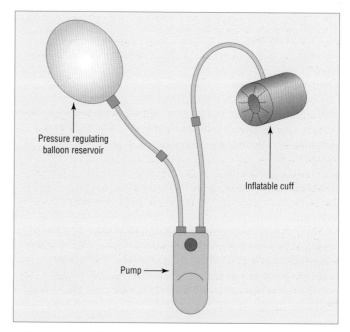

Pressure regulating balloon reservoir

Inflatable cuff

Pump →

Artificial urinary sphincter

The presenting features of vesicovaginal fistula may vary from a watery vaginal discharge to continuous incontinence during the night and day. The appearance of any symptoms of incontinence after recent pelvic surgery should raise suspicion about the development of a vesicovaginal fistula.

A complete examination of the patient is needed to establish the presence of vesicovaginal fistula. Often an acute presentation of a vesicovaginal fistula will be apparent vaginally as an area of inflammation and erythema. A more longstanding fistula may be seen as a small opening in the vaginal wall. On occasions, more than one fistulous track may be present, and the "three swab" test may be useful.

Three swab test for diagnosis of vesicovaginal fistula

- Three separate sponge swabs are placed into the vagina one above the other
- The bladder is then filled with a coloured agent such as methylene blue, and the swabs are removed after 10 minutes
- Discolouration of only the lowest swab suggests that urine has come down the vagina—as a result of a low urethral fistula or from back flow into the introitus
- A ureterovaginal fistula will cause the uppermost swab to become wet but not discoloured, as the urine will have come from the ureter above the level of the bladder
- A vesicovaginal fistula normally is confirmed when the topmost swab is wet and stained blue by fluid leaking from bladder into vagina

---

Radiological imaging with an intravenous urogram is useful to rule out associated ureterovaginal fistulae and also may show obstruction to the ureter or urine extravasation into the retroperitoneum. Cystoscopy and examination under anaesthesia is essential to assess mobility of tissues and to plan any subsequent surgical repair. Retrograde ureterography can also be performed at the same time if the intravenous urogram is unhelpful.

Spontaneous closure of small vesicovaginal fistulae has been reported if the bladder is drained with a catheter, but most patients will need to undergo a surgical repair. A full discussion of the range of operations available is beyond the scope of this chapter, but articles of interest are listed as further reading.

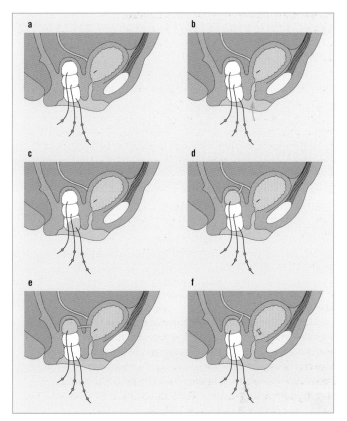

Three swab test. Adapted from Chapple C, Turner Warmick R, *BJU Int* 2005;95:193–214 with permission of the publishers, Blackwell Publishing

---

Further reading

- Abrams P, Blaivas JG, Stanton SL, Andersen JT. The standardization of terminology of lower urinary tract function: report from the standardization subcommittee of the International Continence Society. *Neuro Urol Urodynam* 2002;21;167–78.
- Smith GL, Williams G. Vesicovaginal fistula. *BJU Int* 1999;83:554–70.
- Chapple C, Turner Warwick R. Vesico-vaginal fistula. *BJU Int* 2005;95:193–214.
- Huang WC, Zinman LN, Bihrle W. Surgical repair of vesicovaginal fistulas. *Urol Clin N Am* 2002; 29:709–23.

4   Urological emergencies

Adam Jones

Several urological emergencies can present to medical professionals other than specialist urologists.

Retention of urine

Retention of urine can occur acutely or chronically. Acute retention is characterised by an acute onset of suprapubic discomfort associated with the desire, but inability, to urinate. It is typically seen in men, when the cause is usually obstructive: for example, benign prostatic hyperplasia, prostate cancer, or urethral stricture. It can occur in women, when a pelvic mass should be excluded. Other causes of acute retention are urinary tract infection, constipation, and neurological disorders.

Treatment
Urethral catheterisation is straightforward and will relieve the patient's symptoms instantly. For patients with a history of urethral stricture or previous traumatic catheterisations, however, care needs to be taken. If any resistance is felt, do not persist but seek help from an experienced colleague. Suprapubic catheterisation may be needed.

Clinical course
Acute retention of urine usually occurs in one of two settings:

- Out of the blue— Typically, these patients have little in the way of preceding symptoms in the lower urinary tract and would have a smaller residual volume (perhaps <900 ml). A trial without catheter with or without preceding α blockers may be justified.
- After pre-existing deterioration—Retention merely represents an "end of the road" phenomenon. In this scenario, and certainly in patients with residual volumes much greater than 900 ml, the chance of a long lasting successful trial without catheter is limited, and they should probably proceed to transurethral resection of the prostate.

Chronic urinary retention develops over time and is painless. The classic presentation is in an older man who develops nocturnal enuresis, which occurs as a consequence of overflow and probably is related to relaxation of the resting sphincter pressure during sleep.

Chronic retention can be associated with chronic renal failure. In this case, initial catheterisation is essential; however, it may be followed by postobstructive diuresis, and careful fluid balance will be required if this occurs. Management includes daily monitoring of creatinine and electrolytes, weight, and postural blood pressures. In patients with chronic retention, with or without renal failure, trial without catheter is not appropriate, and patients should proceed to transurethral resection of the prostate if they are medically fit or one of the less invasive alternatives such as laser or microwave prostatectomy. In patients with significant medical problems, options include prostatic stenting, intermittent self-catheterisation, or long term catheterisation.

Renal colic

Renal colic presents with severe pain that often is described as the patient's worst ever pain. Typically, this starts in the flank and radiates around the abdomen, and it can radiate into the testes in men and the labia in women. When a patient describes the position of pain from renal colic, they will adopt a

---

Causes of urinary retention
- Benign prostatic hyperplasia
- Prostatic carcinoma
- Urethral stricture
- Pelvic mass (especially in women)
- Urinary tract infection
- Constipation
- Neurological
- Postoperative pain or immobility

Important points about catheterisation
- Record the volume of urine drained on initial catheterisation (residual urine)
- Catheterisation in the presence of urinary tract infection can precipitate sepsis
- In male trauma patients, consider urethral rupture (blood at the meatus, perineal bruising, and possible high riding prostate)

Predisposing causes of acute urinary retention

Out of the blue	Pre-existing deterioration
• Constipation, postoperative pain, and prolonged car journeys	• Deteriorating lower urinary tract symptoms for some time

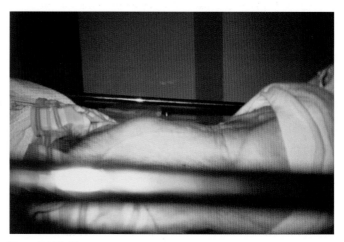

Distended bladder

classic hand position, with their palm overlying the kidney, their fingers pointing posterior, and the thumb pointing anterior down towards the umbilicus.

If a patient uses this classic hand position, this is almost diagnostic of renal colic in itself. Unlike the pain of peritonitis, which is also severe, the patients do not lie still and, typically, are restless and cannot get comfortable in any position.

Abdominal examination is frequently unremarkable, but this may help to exclude other differential diagnoses: for example, acute appendicitis, diverticulitis, salpingitis, and ruptured abdominal aortic aneurysm. If urinalysis does not show microscopic haematuria, an alternative diagnosis should be strongly considered.

Patients should have an intravenous urogram or computed tomography urogram, depending on local preference. The initial management is symptomatic, with analgesics such as diclofenac and antiemetics.

The chances of a renal calculus passing spontaneously largely depend on its size. Calculi <4 mm in size should be treated conservatively, as 90% will pass spontaneously. Fifty per cent of calculi of 4–6 mm will pass spontaneously, but only 10–20% of those >6 mm will pass spontaneously. Intervention thus is required only for stones that are highly unlikely to pass spontaneously, for stones that should pass spontaneously but do not over a period of several weeks, and for those that cause continuous symptoms. Most stones can be treated by extracorporeal shockwave lithotripsy or ureteroscopy and basketing or fragmentation by a variety of methods.

One absolute indication for intervention is the case of an obstructed infected system. Affected patients typically are unwell, with a history of rigors and pyrexia. They need urgent percutaneous nephrostomy, although this intervention itself can precipitate a septic crisis. To avoid missing an obstructed infected system, a diagnosis of "pyelonephritis" should be made in hospital, with an ultrasound or intravenous urogram to exclude obstruction.

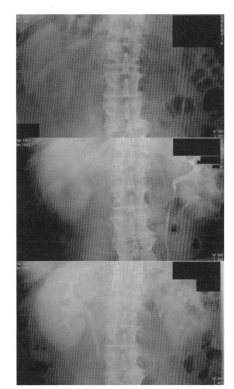

Intravenous urogram showing a 7 mm calculus in the region of the mid-ureter opposite L3 on the control film (top), delayed nephrogram on the right compared with the left (middle), dilated obstructed ureter on later films (bottom)

Conservative management of ureteric calculi

Size of stone (mm)	Management
< 4	Conservative initially as 90 % will pass spontaneously
4–6	50 % pass spontaneously
> 6	Intervention likely as only 10 % will pass spontaneously

Testicular torsion

Any man who presents with an acute onset of testicular pain should be considered as having testicular torsion. The peak age for this is in adolescence; it is rare in men older than 30 years. The main differential diagnoses are torsion of the hydatid of Morgagni (which typically occurs in younger children), epididymitis (which is usually caused by *Chlamydia* in younger men and is related to urinary tract infections in older men), and, rarely, testicular tumours.

Younger children localise pain poorly, so the testes always should be examined—especially in younger children who present with abdominal pain. The classic presentation for testicular torsion is a sudden onset of pain that typically wakes the patient at night and is associated with abdominal discomfort and possibly vomiting.

On examination, the testis is usually very tender and often is riding high or lying abnormally as a result of shortening of the cord via the torsion. The golden rule is that if any doubt exists, the patient should have a scrotal exploration, as the blood supply to the testis is completely cut off in torsion and the testis will die in about six hours.

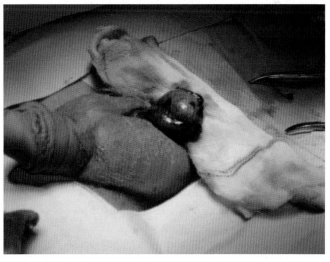

Testicular torsion showing necrosis of affected testis

Priapism

Priapism is characterised by a persistent painful erection unrelated to sexual desire. Priapism may be divided into low flow and high flow. Low flow priapism is a urological emergency, whereas high flow priapism is not. High flow priapism usually has a preceding history of perineal trauma. The aspirated blood also can be sent for blood gas analysis to see if the blood is arterial or venous in origin. Oral terbutaline may also be helpful, especially in the primary care setting. Other conservative measures may be successful, such as asking the patient to climb the stairs (the "arterial steal" syndrome) or applying ice packs.

If these measures fail and, certainly if the erection has been present for more than four hours, the patient should be reviewed in hospital and the corpora should be aspirated with a butterfly needle and syringe. This is done on the lateral aspect of the penis to avoid the neurovascular bundles dorsally and the urethra ventrally. If this fails, slow infusion of an α agonist such as phenylephrine is the next step unless the initial aspiration reveals bright red blood, which would suggest a penile arteriovenous shunt. If this still fails, the patient will need surgery, starting with a Winter shunt to create communication between the corpora cavernosa and corpus spongiosum of the glans penis.

Paraphimosis

Paraphimosis is swelling of the glans penis and a failure of the foreskin to protract over the glans having been previously retracted. It usually occurs in the setting of a mild phimosis, where the foreskin is a little tight.

Most commonly, it occurs in elderly catheterised patients or in younger men after an early sexual experience. The tight retracted foreskin causes the glans to swell, with subsequent swelling of the foreskin itself.

To reduce the foreskin, the oedema needs to be squeezed out of the glans penis by gentle but persistent pressure on the glans for several minutes. This can be helped by using a penile ring block with 1% plain lignocaine. Once the size of the glans is reduced, the retracted foreskin can be pulled back to its normal position. Should this procedure fail, the patient will need to have the restricting "ring" of the prepuce incised under a general anaesthetic, which will allow the foreskin to be pulled forward again. Elective circumcision almost always should be performed several weeks later.

Spinal cord compression

Spinal cord compression is an acute medical emergency. It often presents to urologists because metastatic prostate cancer is one of the most common causes.

Symptoms often are rapidly progressive and irreversible, so prompt diagnosis is essential. Unfortunately, the classic presentation is rather non-specific, with the patient often described as "off his legs".

Perianal sensation often is the first sensation lost, and this can be associated with loss of the bulbocavernosal reflex. This reflex is seen visually as contraction of the anus on stroking the perianal skin or squeezing the glans penis. Decreased anal tone may be associated with this. An urgent magnetic resonance scan is the investigation of choice, and, if spinal cord compression is confirmed, urgent neurological advice should be sought. Intravenous corticosteroids should be given and urgent spinal decompression or radiotherapy performed.

In patients with cord compression secondary to prostate cancer who are not already on hormone ablation, this may also be a case for an emergency orchidectomy.

Some causes of priapism
- Intracavernosal pharmacotherapy for erectile dysfunction
- Leukaemia, sickle cell disease, or pelvic tumour
- Penile or spinal cord trauma
- Idiopathic causes

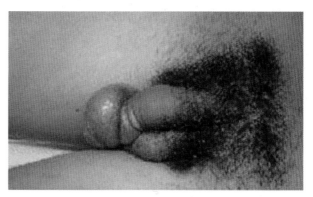

Paraphimosis

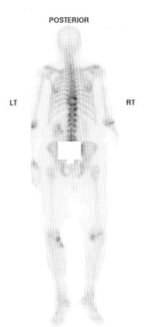

Isotope bone scan with thoracic and lumbar metastases

Specific symptoms of spinal cord compression to elicit
- Altered sensation or paraesthesia in legs
- Leg weakness or difficulty walking
- Urinary incontinence or retention
- Faecal incontinence

Associated with these symptoms may be signs of:
- Decreased muscle tone in the lower limbs
- Reduced power
- Abnormal sensation
- "Sensory level:" this is shown by "wiggling" an examining finger down the patient's midline starting at the jugular notch and moving inferiorly. The sensory level at which the patient notices a change in sensation corresponds roughly to the level at which the spinal cord compression is present

Top 10 tips for urological emergencies

- If urethral catheterisation is not straightforward, do not force it—seek experienced help.
- Always record the immediate post-catheterisation residual volume, as this may influence subsequent management
- If an older patient develops nocturnal enuresis, always suspect chronic retention.
- In patients with pelvic trauma, remember the possibility of a ruptured urethra.
- Obstruction and infection in a kidney are urological emergencies.
- Beware renal colic on the left side in older men—consider a ruptured abdominal aortic aneurysm
- Any testicular pain in a young man is torsion until proved otherwise.
- Priapism needs to be corrected rapidly to avoid ischaemic fibrosis of the penis.
- Do not rush paraphimosis reduction. Persistent pressure is needed on the swollen glans for several minutes to decompress it.
- Do not forget spinal cord compression in a patient with a known primary cancer that has a strong tendency to metastasise to the bone (prostate and kidney, as well as breast, bronchus, and thyroid).

Further reading

- Jones A, Turner K, Handa A. Surgical emergencies:urological emergencies. *Student BMJ* 2000;8:268–269.
- Rosenstein D., McAninch JW. Urologic emergencies. *Med Clin North Am* 2004;88:495–518.
- Keoghane SR, Sullivan ME, Miller MA. The aetiology, pathogenesis and management of priapism. *BJU Int* 2002;90:149–154.
- Reynard JM, Barua JM. Reduction of paraphimosis the simple way—the Dundee technique. *BJU Int* 1999;83:859–860.
- Shah J, Whitfield HN. Urolithiasis through the ages. *BJU Int* 2002;89:801–810.

The photograph showing paraphimosis is with permission from Raynard JM. *BJU Int* 1999;83:859–600.

5 Subfertility and male sexual dysfunction

Stephanie Symons

Subfertility

Subfertility is defined as failure to conceive after regular unprotected sexual intercourse over a period of one year. About 15% of couples are thought to be affected by infertility: 50% as a result of factors in the woman, 20% as a result of factors in the man and 30% as a result of factors in the man and woman. This chapter considers only male subfertility.

Male fertility is a complex process that requires an intact endocrine axis, successful spermatogenesis, satisfactory sperm delivery to the woman's genital tract, and sperm capable of penetrating the woman's ova. The causes for male subfertility are numerous and can affect any one of these processes. Clinical assessment of subfertile men is aimed at identifying any reversible cause for subfertility and excluding significant underlying pathology. Assessment should also identify causes of subfertility that are suitable for treatment with assisted reproductive techniques. In cases of subfertility that are not reversible or cannot be managed by assisted reproductive techniques, artificial insemination by donor sperm or adoption can be advised.

Initial assessment of subfertile men must include careful history, physical examination, and semen analysis. A sexual history provides details of erectile or ejaculatory dysfunction and abstinence. Past medical and surgical history should elucidate previous genitourinary infections and trauma, as well as cryptorchidism or torsion. Attention should also be paid to the use of drugs and the woman's reproductive history. General physical examination may give clues to an underlying chromosomal abnormality, and examination of the genitals can identify hypogonadism, absent testes or vas deferens, and penile anomalies such as hypospadias and chordee.

Semen analysis is the cornerstone of the assessment of subfertile men. Semen should be produced by masturbation after three days of abstinence and must be examined within two hours of collection. Two separate samples are usually analysed, and, in most cases, the results of semen analysis guide further investigation and treatment.

Subfertile men should be managed further by a multidisciplinary team in specialist fertility centres at which cryopreservation of sperm is available. Men with normal results after semen analysis may need to be counselled about the timing of intercourse and avoidance of lubricants. The female partners of normospermic men may need further evaluation.

In men with an absent or low volume ejaculate, the question is whether the patient has retrograde ejaculation, obstructed ejaculatory ducts, or failure of emission. In the absence of obstructed ejaculatory ducts, azoospermic men with testicular failure or absent vas deferens will need genetic counselling about chromosomal abnormalities. Reduced numbers of sperm, known as oligospermia, is an indication for hormone studies. Levels of testosterone, follicle stimulating hormone, and luteinising hormone should be checked in men with <5–10 million sperm/ml to exclude a treatable endocrine cause. A diagnosis of primary testicular failure may also be established.

If further assessment by testicular biopsy is required, some sperm should be cryopreserved, as this avoids a second operation to retrieve sperm if assisted reproduction is to be undertaken. Varicocelectomy and antisperm antibody testing are not advised, as no evidence shows that varicocelectomy

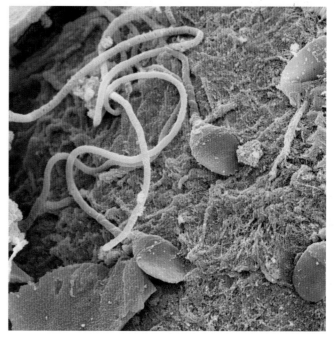

Spermatozoa penetrating an ovum during fertilisation. With permission from Eye of Science/Science Photo Library

---

Causes of male factor infertility

Endocrine disorders

- Pituitary disease
- Hypogonadotropic hypogonadism
- Excess of androgens

Disorders of spermatogenesis

- Chromosomal disorders
- Cryptorchidism
- Testicular torsion
- Sertoli cell only
- Infection

Sperm delivery disorders

- Congenital bilateral absence of vas deferens
- Ductal obstruction
- Erectile dysfunction
- Ejaculatory dysfunction

Penile anatomical disorders

Sperm function disorders

- Immunological infertility
- Ultrastructural abnormalities of sperm

WHO criteria for normal seminal fluid analysis (2002)

- Volume > 2 ml
- Sperm concentration > 20 million/ml
- Sperm motility > 50% progressive or > 25% rapidly progressive
- Morphology (strict criteria) > 15% normal forms
- Vitality > 75% live
- White blood cells < 1 million/ml

increases male fertility and no treatment is effective against antisperm antibodies. If varicocelectomy is required, this may be performed by open ligation, laparoscopic ligation, or radiological embolisation.

Assisted reproductive techniques have revolutionised the treatment of couples affected by subfertility. Intrauterine injection of sperm can be used in men with problems with delivery of sperm into the woman's reproductive tract, such as retrograde ejaculation and severe hypospadias. In vitro fertilisation is used in combination with female superovulation and ova harvesting when reasonable volumes of good quality sperm can be extracted from the man. Fertile sperm are retrieved from the epididymis in such men by microsurgical or percutaneous sperm aspiration—percutaneous epididymal sperm extraction or testicular sperm extraction. In cases of severe male factor subfertility, however, intracytoplasmic sperm injection has become the technique of choice.

Intracytoplasmic sperm injection involves the injection of a single spermatozoon into an ovum retrieved for in vitro fertilisation. A single spermatozoon can be harvested in nearly all men from the epididymis or testis, even in cases of testicular failure. Most couples affected by severe male factor subfertility can therefore now be treated with intracytoplasmic sperm injection. Factors that relate to the woman, such as age, have a considerable impact on the success rates of intracytoplasmic sperm injection, which have been recorded as up to 33%.

Erectile dysfunction

The subcellular understanding of erectile function has produced a revolution in its treatment. From a vascular standpoint, normal male erection depends on three integrated processes:

- Arterial inflow to the penis increases, filling the sinusoids of the corpora cavernosa
- Cavernosal smooth muscle relaxation aids arterial inflow
- Subsequent compression and elongation of the subtunical veins drain the corpora cavernosa decrease venous outflow and aid rigidity.

Evaluation of men with erectile dysfunction must include a careful history to elucidate psychogenic causes. Risk factors for cardiovascular disease are also now known to be the most important risk factors for physiological erectile dysfunction. Patients should be advised to stop smoking and should undergo screening for hypertension, hypercholesterolaemia, diabetes, and renal disease. Hormone evaluation should include early morning free testosterone in patients with diminished sexual interest or suspected hypogonadism. In patients with low levels of testosterone, the results should be confirmed and luteinising hormone, follicle stimulating hormone, and prolactin should be assessed to exclude prolactinoma before secondary referral.

Oral agents for erectile dysfunction have reduced the urologist's role in this area. Most patients with erectile dysfunction can now be treated within the community with one of the phosphodiesterase inhibitors. These drugs differ from each other in terms of onset of action and half life, but their efficacy seems to be equal.

Patients should be advised to take phosphodiesterase inhibitors about one hour before sexual intercourse is desired, although some drugs, such as tadalafil, may produce potency over a much longer period. Sexual stimulation is needed to potentiate the effect of these drugs, and failure to respond to them often is a result of a lack of understanding of this fact. Initial failure should not be an endpoint in itself, and the patient should be encouraged to try again on up to five or six occasions, with increasing doses of drugs where appropriate.

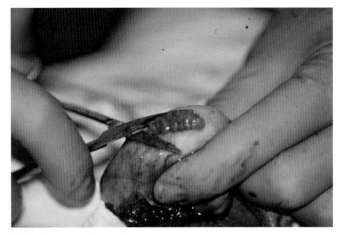

Testicular exploration and sperm extraction

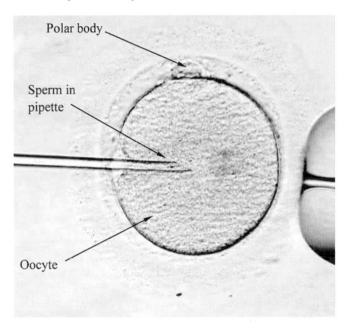

Intracytoplasmic sperm injection. Reproduced from Braude P, Rowell P. Assisted conception. In Braude P, Taylor A (eds). *ABC of subfertility*. Oxford: Blackwell Publishing, 2004.

Risk factors for erectile dysfunction

Most important risk factors	Additional risk factors
• Age	• Psychological factors
• Cardiovascular disease	• Trauma
• Hyperlipidaemia	• Pelvic surgery
• Diabetes mellitus	• Neurological disorders
• Drug side effects	• Hormonal disorders
• Smoking	• Excessive alcohol

Comparisons of phosphodiesterase inhibitors

Variable	Sildenafil	Tadalafil	Vardenafil
T_{max} (hours)	1	2	< 1
T1/2 (hours)	3–5	17.5	3–5
Onset of action (minutes)	30–60	30–45	20–45
Duration (hours)	4	> 24	4
Metabolism	Hepatic	Hepatic	Hepatic
Side effects	Headache, facial flushing, dyspepsia, nasal congestion	Headache, facial flushing, dyspepsia, nasal congestion	Headache, facial flushing, dyspepsia, nasal congestion

It may also be useful to try more than one phosphodiesterase inhibitor before deciding that the drugs are not going to be of benefit.

The drug of choice is determined by individual patient preference. Phosphodiesterase inhibitors are contraindicated in patients who are using nitrates, because of the risk of profound hypotension. Patients with intermediate or high risk cardiac status should be referred to a cardiologist before their erectile dysfunction is treated. Patients who do not respond to phosphodiesterase inhibitors should have the opportunity to see a urologist.

Patients who fail on oral treatments for erectile dysfunction can be treated with intracavernosal pharmacotherapy, a vacuum device, or insertion of a penile prosthesis. Intracavernosal injection of prostaglandin E_1 remains one of the most reliable ways of gaining an erection, although many patients find self-injection disagreeable. The use of a vacuum device is less invasive than intracavernosal injection. For patients who will not respond to other treatment for erectile dysfunction, a penile prosthesis is considered. Prostheses can be divided into malleable, inflatable, or non-inflatable types. Insertion of a prosthesis requires strict asepsis under a general anaesthetic, and infection remains the most important complication. An infected penile prosthesis should be removed.

Vacuum device

- Patient places flaccid penis into device
- Air is withdrawn, creating a vacuum that draws blood into the penis and results in an erection
- Erection is maintained by placing constriction band around the base of the penis

Peyronie's disease

The symptomatic incidence of Peyronie's disease is thought to be 1%. Affected men present with pain and deformity on erection, a palpable penile plaque, and, in many cases, erectile dysfunction. Peyronie's disease is associated with Dupuytren's contracture and a history of penile trauma. Minor injury to the tunica albuginea is thought to lead to trapping of fibrin and an excess cytokine reaction that causes disordered healing and focal loss of elasticity. Clinically, the disease undergoes acute and chronic phases. During the acute phase, which can last up to two years, the erectile deformity may worsen, so it is important to resist surgical intervention during this time.

Various medical treatments have been tried for Peyronie's disease, but none has been shown to be effective, although patients may ask to try one of these.

In patients whose deformity prevents intercourse, surgical intervention is needed. The penile curvature is corrected by excision and plication of the contralateral tunica (Nesbitt procedure) or excision and grafting at the plaque site (Lue procedure). The Nesbitt operation causes penile shortening, while the Lue procedure risks erectile dysfunction.

Treatments tried in patients with Peyronie's disease

- Extracorporeal shock wave lithotripsy
- Injections of verapamil
- Vitamin E therapy
- Para-aminobenzoate tablets

Intracavernosal injection of prostaglandin E_1

- Once the correct dose is established by titration against the desired effect, the patient is taught good injection technique
- The injection is placed laterally into the base of the penis, avoiding the urethra ventrally and the neurovascular bundle dorsally
- Complications including pain and fibrosis at the injection site and priapism should be outlined to the patient

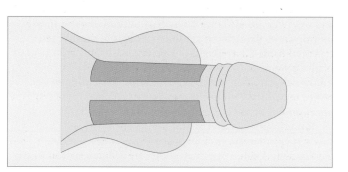

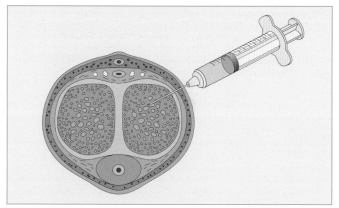

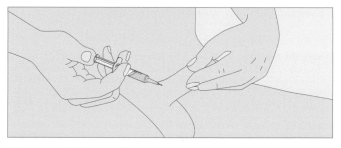

Intracavernosal pharmacotherapy

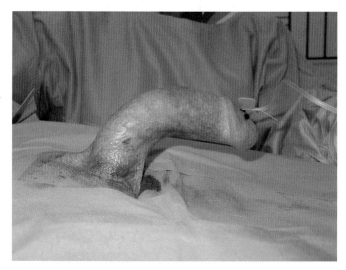

Curvature of penis in Peyronie's disease

The ageing male

In recent years, interest has grown in the concept of androgen decline in the ageing male, which is known as "andropause." Androgen decline in the ageing male is relatively common, and the cause is thought to be multifactorial. It is characterised by reduced levels of androgen in the serum, with or without changes in androgen receptor sensitivity. Androgen deficiency can affect multiple organ systems and result in significant reduction in quality of life, including sexual function. Clinically, it is important to differentiate between the ageing male who has symptomatic hypogonadism, who may require treatment, and the ageing male without symptoms, who does not. Symptomatic patients with low levels of testosterone in serum can be treated with a variety of forms of testosterone to maintain levels within the physiological range. Liver function, lipids, and levels of prostate specific antigen should be monitored regularly in patients started on androgen replacement therapy. Androgens are absolutely contraindicated in men with definite or suspected prostate or breast cancer.

The diagrams showing the technique for intracavernosal pharmacotherapy were adapted from a leaflet published by Pharmacia and Upjohn. The photograph showing testicular exploration and sperm extraction is courtesy of Suks Minhas, and the photograph of Peyronie's disease is courtesy of Mr David Ralph.

Clinical picture of androgen decline in ageing men

- Decreased sexual desire and erectile quality
- Decreased intellectual capacity (depression or fatigue)
- Decreased lean body mass
- Decreased bone mineral density
- Decreased body hair and skin alterations
- Decreased visceral fat
- Increase in abnormal sleep patterns

Further reading

- National Institute for Clinical Excellence. *Fertility:assessment and treatment for people with fertility problems.* London: National Institute for Clinical Excellence, 2004. Available at http://www.nice.org.uk/pdf/CG011fullguideline.pdf (last accessed 24 Jan 2006).
- American Urological Association. *Erectile dysfunction. The management of erectile dysfunction: an update.* American Urologoical Association, 2005. Available at: www.auanet.org/guidelines/edmgmt.cfm (last accessed 24 Jan 2005).
- Urciuoli R, Cantisani TA, Carlinil M. Prostaglandin E1 for treatment of erectile dysfunction. *Cochrane Library.* Issue 2. Oxford: Update Software, 2005.
- Morales A, Morley JE, Heaton JPW. Practical approach to andropause (ADAM) and androgen therapy. Presented at the 99th Annual Meeting of the American Urological Association, San Francisco, CA, 8–13 May 2004.

6 Management of urinary tract infection in adults

Philippa Cheetham

Definitions

Urinary tract infection is bacterial invasion of the urothelium that results in an inflammatory response. A complicated urinary infection carries a moderate to high risk of sepsis, with significant morbidity and mortality. Risk factors for this should alert the doctor to an increased risk of severe or complicated infection. Bacteriuria is a bacterial urinary tract infection that occurs without any of the usual symptoms. Antibiotic resistance is increasing, so sensitivities should be confirmed on cultures from midstream urine samples.

Common urinary bacterial pathogens

Most urinary infection is ascending. Bowel organisms, which colonise the perineum, displace commensal organisms and ascend into the bladder. The number of bacteria in the bladder is critical to the development of urinary tract infections. Most bacteria are Gram negative bacilli. *Escherichia coli* is the most common organism in both sexes. In young women, *Staphylococcus saprophyticus* is the second most common urinary pathogen and is almost always related to sexual activity.

Bacterial adherence

The process of bacterial cell adhesion is the key to urinary tract infection. Bacterial adhesins produced by pili on the bacterial surface are important in pathogenesis: for example, the P fimbriae possessed by *E coli*. The specific adhesins determine the degree and site of invasion. Adhesion of bacteria to the epithelium is followed by proliferation, invasion, and initiation of the inflammatory process. Protective glycoprotein layers that cover the urothelium are broken down, promoting colonisation of the exposed deeper layers. Patients susceptible to urinary tract infection also have increased carriage of adhesive bacteria in the large intestine, perineum, introitus, and prepuce.

Management of urinary tract infection in women

Urinary tract infection is extremely common in women, as the short urethral length permits easy bacterial colonisation of the bladder. At least 20% of women can expect to experience a urinary tract infection in their lifetime.

Diagnosis and investigation

Infection of the lower urinary tract may be diagnosed by dipstick urine analysis. The dipstick is frequently positive for blood because of inflammation of the bladder wall. The leucocyte esterase test detects pus cells in the urine. Bacteria in the urine that reduce nitrate to nitrite are detected by the nitrate reductase test. Protein is also often detected.

Reasons for negative culture from midstream urine in presence of cystitis symptoms

Sterile urine

- Irritative symptoms not due to infection

Infected urine

- Urinary dilution following high fluid intake
- Specimen collection in early stages of urinary tract infection
- Infection partially treated with antibiotics
- Specimen stored for too long so organisms not cultured

Features of urinary tract infections

- Urinary tract infection is common, particularly in women
- Urinary tract infection may be less common in men because the extra urethral length prevents bacterial colonisation of the bladder
- Cystitis produces symptoms of frequency, urgency, dysuria, and suprapubic pain
- Local symptoms may be absent, particularly in elderly people, who may present only with increasing confusion
- Urine often has an offensive odour
- Underlying functional or anatomic disorders must be excluded
- Ascending infection causes pyelonephritis, which typically presents with fever, loin pain, and malaise

---

Risk factors for complicated urinary tract infection

- Male sex
- Old age
- Febrile urinary tract infection
- Symptoms for > 7 days
- Haematuria
- History of stone disease
- Recent hospitalisation
- Urinary tract instrumentation
- Pregnancy
- Diabetes
- Immunosuppression
- Infection with drug resistant organism
- Functional or structural abnormality

Common urinary bacterial pathogens

- *Escherichia coli*
- *Staphylococcus saprophyticus*
- *Streptococcus faecalis*
- *Proteus* spp
- *Pseudomonas* spp
- *Klebsiella* spp
- *Providencia* spp
- *Citrobacter* spp
- *Serratia* spp
- *Enterococcus faecalis*

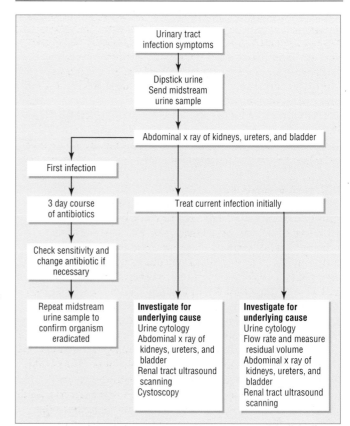

Diagnosis and investigation of urinary tract infections

A midstream urine sample should be sent for microscopy and culture to confirm the presence of bacteria and pyuria. The midstream urine sample should thus be collected before antibiotics are started. The laboratory will also test for sensitivity to antibiotics.

Once the infection has been treated, a repeat midstream urine sample should be sent for culture to confirm that the organism has been eradicated. If haematuria persists after the infection has been treated. this should be investigated accordingly.

Single episodes of documented infection in otherwise normal women need no special investigations, but repeated episodes of cystitis in women need to be investigated. Regular urine cultures will help identify women with abacterial cystitis, as well as differentiating those with recurrent bacterial cystitis, which is the result of bacterial persistence or reinfection. Reinfection is responsible for > 95% of recurrent urinary tract infections in women. An on demand facility for midstream urine samples, at which the patient can drop in a urine sample to the general practice when they are symptomatic, will increase the success of accurate categorisation.

Cystoscopy—with a flexible scope using local anaesthetic or rigid cystoscopy under general anaesthetic—permits visualisation of the bladder wall. A plain x ray of the kidneys, ureters, and bladder and a renal ultrasound examination will exclude upper tract abnormalities including stones. An ultrasound of the bladder combined with uroflowmetry will detect a residual volume and show the flow rate profile. A tight urethral meatus in women can result in poor bladder drainage and urinary infection. When obstructive symptoms predominate, a cystoscopy and urethral dilatation may improve flow and prevent further infection.

Treatment

Uncomplicated urinary tract infections usually respond to a course of three days of oral antibiotics. Patient compliance with respect to completing the course at the correct dose maximises treatment success and minimises development of resistance. If urinary tract infections are related to sexual activity, a single dose of an antibiotic may be taken after sexual intercourse. Long term low dose antibiotic prophylaxis is an option for those who continue to suffer recurrent attacks despite taking preventative measures.

Prevention

Prevention is better than cure. Lifestyle advice should be given to reduce the frequency of attacks.

Differential diagnosis

Other inflammatory conditions that give rise to a similar symptom complex of frequency, urgency, dysuria, and suprapubic pain can be misdiagnosed as recurrent lower urinary tract infections. Patients who present with persistent symptoms or no growth on urine culture should therefore be referred to a urologist for further investigation. In both men and women, the possibility of bladder carcinoma mimicking symptoms of infection should be excluded by urine cytology analysis, as well as cystoscopy and biopsy if necessary. Other inflammatory conditions include trigonitis and interstitial cystitis. The midstream urine sample is usually free of infection, although infection can coexist. The trigone at the base of the bladder is oestrogen dependant. In perimenopausal or postmenopausal women, inflammation of the trigone as a result of hormonal deficiency can result in irritative symptoms that mimic urinary infection. The trigone seems inflamed on cystoscopy, but the rest of the bladder has a normal appearance.

Midstream urine samples

- True urinary tract infections, rather than contaminations, are present with $> 10^5$ bacterial forming colonies/ml of midstream urine
- Many patients with infective urinary symptoms have lower counts
- Presence of more than one type of organism suggests contamination

---

Antibiotic sensitivity testing

- This is becoming increasingly important as the number of resistant organisms increases
- If bacteria present on urine culture are not sensitive to the antibiotic initially prescribed, an alternative needs to be prescribed
- Local knowledge of the bacterial uropathogens and their sensitivity is crucial to minimising the likelihood of prescribing an ineffective antibiotic

---

Categories of women with cystitis symptoms according to bacterial presence

- Bacteria always present in urine
- Bacteria sometimes present in urine
- Bacteria never present in urine

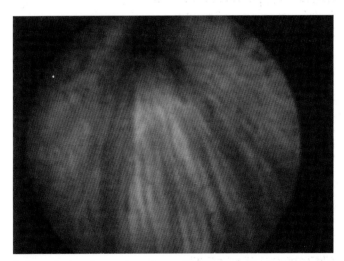

Endoscopic view of prostatic urethra and bladder neck. Provided by Mr H N Blackford

---

Prevention of urinary tract infections in women

- Maintaining adequate fluid intake
- Ensuring that bladder is fully empty
- Emptying bladder before and after sexual intercourse
- Avoiding constipation
- Wearing cotton underwear
- Avoid using vaginal deodorants and perfumed toiletries in baths
- Rubber diaphragms and some spermicidal creams can aggravate symptoms
- Cranberry juice may have a definite antibacterial effect

Pregnancy

Pregnancy is associated with bacteriuria, so symptomatic urinary tract infection is common. Hormones of pregnancy cause ureteric relaxation. Pressure of the fetal head in the pelvis compresses the ureters, with physiological hydronephrosis almost inevitable as pregnancy progresses. Urinary alkalinity, which would encourage growth of Gram negative organisms, may also be a relevant predisposing factor to urinary tract infection in pregnancy. Ascending infection that results in acute pyelonephritis can thus easily occur. Urinary infection therefore should be taken seriously in pregnancy, as it can result in premature delivery and perinatal mortality. Women are screened for bacteriuria at the first prenatal visit and throughout pregnancy. If present, it should be treated with antibiotics that are not contraindicated in pregnancy.

Management of urinary tract infections in men

Urinary tract infection is less common in men. A single urinary tract infection needs full investigation, as described for women. Recurrent infection is more commonly the result of bacterial persistence than reinfection. Prostatitis and epididymo-orchitis can be associated with urinary tract infections in men and often require a prolonged course of antibiotics (4–6 weeks). Digital rectal examination to assess for a tender painful prostate, as well as examination of the external genitalia to assess for tenderness of the testes and epididymi, should therefore always be performed in men.

Upper urinary tract infection

Acute pyelonephritis is defined as inflammation of the renal parenchyma and renal pelvis. The diagnosis is usually made clinically on the basis of loin pain, fever, chills, and general malaise. Vomiting is not uncommon. Lower urinary tract symptoms may be minimal at presentation. If the patient is pyrexial, blood cultures should be arranged as well as urine cultures. Prompt renal ultrasound imaging should be performed primarily to exclude obstruction. Anatomical abnormalities and renal stones may be detected. Intravenous urogram or computed tomography are alternative investigations. Treatment includes intravenous antibiotics, intravenous hydration, analgesia, and an antiemetic if necessary. Intravenous antibiotics are usually given for 24–48 hours. Oral antibiotics should then be continued for 10–14 days. The patient may take several weeks to return to normal health.

Infection in presence of obstructed upper tract

An infected obstructed upper urinary tract is a urological emergency and is potentially life threatening. If this is confirmed on imaging, prompt decompression is essential. Percutaneous drainage of the kidney under local anaesthetic with a nephrostomy tube can be performed in the radiology department. Alternatively, retrograde placement of a ureteric stent can be done in theatre. In ill patients, nephrostomy drainage is preferable. The cause of obstruction can be dealt with at a later date, when the sepsis has resolved and the patient is well again.

Causes of urinary tract infections in men

- Local obstructive causes including urethral stricture, high bladder neck and an obstructive prostate can be detected at flexible cystoscopy.
- Urethrotomy, bladder neck incision or transurethral resection of the prostate can be arranged respectively if necessary.
- Bladder stones form in stagnant urine, when obstruction prevents drainage. They can often be detected with a KUB x-ray. Cystoscopy will also reveal if bladder stones are present. Stones cause infection and infection can exacerbate further stone infection.
- Transrectal prostate needle biopsy carries a risk of complications, including urinary tract infection. Prophylactic antibiotics pre and post biopsy are given to reduce the risk of bacteraemia resulting in life threatening sepsis.

> The only two antibiotics to penetrate the prostate are trimethoprim and ciprofloxacin, which should be remembered when the most appropriate antibiotic is selected in men with urinary tract infections

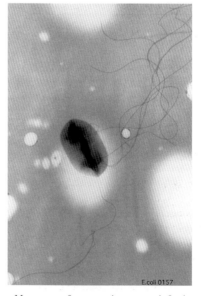

E.coli 0157

Most cases of upper urinary tract infection are caused by Gram negative bacteria, predominantly *Escherichia coli*. Courtesy of CDC/Peggy S Hayes

7 Prostate cancer

Chris Dawson

Epidemiology

Prostate cancer is the most common cancer in men in the United Kingdom and accounts for 20% of cancers in men overall but only 13% of deaths from cancer in men. Survival at five years in men diagnosed with prostate cancer in England and Wales has more than doubled in the last 20 years.

The risk of developing prostate cancer is linked to age, and most cases are diagnosed in men aged 70–79 years. The stage at presentation has changed dramatically over the last 20 years, with more cases being localised at presentation.

Symptoms and signs

Early prostate cancer produces no specific symptoms, so most men present with lower urinary tract symptoms of benign prostatic hyperplasia (see Chapter 2). About 10% of patients who undergo surgery for benign prostatic hyperplasia will be found to have prostate cancer after histological examination of the prostate.

Investigation

Men referred with lower urinary tract symptoms should undergo a full history and clinical examination. The latter should always include digital rectal examination of the prostate.

The use of levels of prostate specific antigen has led to more frequent diagnosis of early prostate cancer. Considerable debate surrounds its use in patients with suspected prostate cancer, as the overall accuracy of the test varies between 64% and 90% in published studies.

Many urological departments have started to use age specific reference ranges for levels of prostate specific antigen rather than absolute cut-off values for normal or abnormal levels. Use of these age specific reference ranges may detect prostate cancer at an early stage in younger men and reduce the number of unnecessary biopsies in older men.

The standard test for prostate specific antigen measures the total amount of the antigen in the bloodstream, but it exists in different states. Most prostate specific antigen in serum is bound to protein, but a proportion exists free in the bloodstream. The proportion of free prostate specific antigen reduces in patients with prostate cancer. The proportion of free prostate specific antigen can be measured, and this can be expressed as a ratio of the level of total prostate specific antigen. A free to total prostate specific antigen ratio of < 25% in men with a total level of 4–10 ng/ml has been shown to detect 95% of cancers while avoiding 20% of unnecessary biopsies.

Similarly, the amount of prostate specific antigen bound to protein (complexed prostate specific antigen) can be measured. Complexed prostate specific antigen is more stable in extracted blood samples and may give more reliable results than levels of free prostate specific antigen.

Age specific reference values for prostate specific antigen

Age (years)	40–49	50–59	60–69	70–79
Value (ng/ml)	<2.5	<3.5	<4.5	<6.5

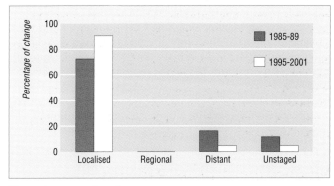

Change in presentation of prostate cancer

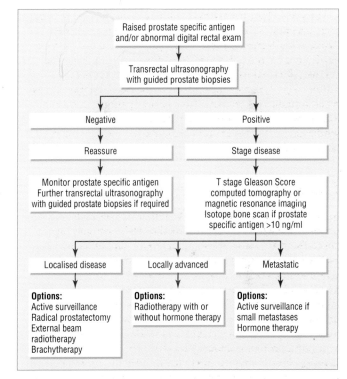

Diagnosis and management of prostate cancer

Counselling patients who request a prostate specific antigen test

- Although the test for prostate specific antigen itself is innocuous, the consequences of an increased level of prostate specific antigen may be more considerable
- A level of prostate specific antigen higher than the age specific reference range requires a transrectal ultrasound and biopsy of the prostate, as long as no contraindications exist
- The biopsy procedure has known complications of haematuria, haemospermia, and rectal bleeding. Important complications, including septicaemia, have been reported but are rare
- A biopsy positive for cancer will lead to a discussion about treatment options for prostate cancer
- A negative biopsy does **not** exclude prostate cancer, and the patient will often need further surveillance of their levels of prostate specific antigen and biopsies later if the levels should rise further

The indications for transrectal ultrasound and biopsy of the prostate are an abnormal finding on digital rectal examination of the prostate or an increased level of prostate specific antigen.

Role of screening for prostate cancer

Although screening with prostate specific antigen for prostate cancer has not been adopted in the United Kingdom, this test remains an important diagnostic tool in many cases. In men who present without lower urinary tract symptoms, the patient must be counselled fully before the test for prostate specific antigen is performed.

A recent review of screening for prostate cancer concluded that prostate cancer remains a major health problem but:

- The natural history is unknown
- The screening test is inefficient
- No agreement exists about effective treatment
- Screening may lead to a reduction in quality of life
- Screening has not been proved to reduce mortality from prostate cancer
- Radical treatment may incur risks and long term side effects
- Whether screening is cost effective is unknown.

Management of prostate cancer

Staging prostate cancer

Before a decision can be made about management, the cancer must be staged with the TNM classification system and given a Gleason score. Most prostate cancers are heterogeneous, and various degrees of histological differentiation will be seen down the microscope. The two most common patterns are given a score of 1 to 5 (with 5 being the most poorly differentiated). This is expressed most commonly as, for example, "Gleason 4 + 3." These values are added together to give a Gleason sum score, which would be "7" in the example above.

Computed tomography and magnetic resonance imaging are often used to stage prostate cancer in order to determine the presence of extracapsular spread or distant metastasis, which might preclude intervention with radical therapy.

Studies, however, have shown that these imaging methods may be of limited value. The resolution of computed tomography is too low to be able to distinguish abnormalities within the prostate gland, the state of the prostatic capsule, or the presence or absence of disease outside the prostate gland. Magnetic resonance imaging seems to be of limited value overall in clinically localised prostate cancer. The use of an endorectal magnetic resonance coil can help predict extracapsular penetration or involvement of the seminal vesicles. Computed tomography and magnetic resonance imaging, however, may have a role in evaluating the status of lymph nodes in patients at risk of involvement of the lymph nodes, who are suitable for radical surgery or radiotherapy.

An isotope bone scan should be performed to exclude metastases in patients who are undergoing radical therapy, in those with a Gleason sum score ≥7, or when a clinical suspicion of metastases exists. Most doctors would omit such a scan in patients with a level of prostate specific antigen <10 ng/ml and a Gleason sum score <7.

Localised prostate cancer

Active surveillance

Active surveillance preserves quality of life by the avoidance of significant complications associated with other treatments. This

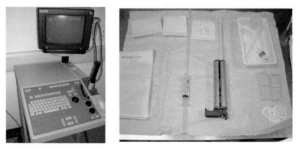

Transrectal ultrasound scan showing prostate cancer (arrow) bulging anteriorly through prostate capsule

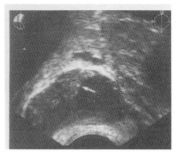

Transrectal ultrasonography machine (left) and biopsy equipment (right). The biopsy gun is designed to be operated one-handed and features an integral safety device to prevent accidental firing. Also shown in the figure is local anaesthetic ready to inject around the prostate using a spinal needle. The use of cassettes (shown in yellow to right of picture) and sponges to transport the biopsies in formalin greatly assists the pathology staff

TNM classification for prostate cancer

Classification	Explanation
T0	No evidence of primary tumour
T1	Tumour is neither palpable nor visible by imaging
T1a	Tumour in < 5% prostate chips at transurethral resection of the prostate
T1b	Tumour in > 5% prostate chips at transurethral resection of the prostate
T1c	Tumour found at prostate biopsy or detected through levels of prostate specific antigen
T2	Palpable tumour or visible on transrectal ultrasound
T2a	Involves one lobe
T2b	Involves both lobes
T3	Tumour extends through prostatic capsule
T3a	Involves one or both sides
T3b	Involves seminal vesicles

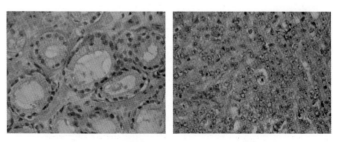

Gleason 3 pattern of prostate cancer (magnification × 20) (left) and Gleason 5 pattern of prostate cancer (×20) (right). Note the marked cytological atypia, nuclear pleomorphism, and lack of gland formation compared with the Gleason 3 pattern

may be suitable for patients at low risk (low levels of prostate specific antigen, low Gleason sum score, and stage T1 or T2). Patients are seen in the outpatient department at intervals of three to six months and are monitored through levels of prostate specific antigen. If the time to doubling of levels of prostate specific antigen is less than three years or if the patient has any signs of clinical progression, active treatment should be pursued. Newer strategies for active surveillance include repeat biopsies every two years if radical treatments are still appropriate.

Radical prostatectomy
Radical prostatectomy has advanced considerably in the last few years, but it remains a procedure with important potential complications, particularly erectile dysfunction, which has been reported in 10–80% of cases. Most surgeons now use a "nerve sparing" approach to dissection around the prostate to maximise the chance of potency. Incontinence is much less of a problem after radical surgery compared with external beam radiotherapy, but it may occur in up to 15% of cases.

External beam radiotherapy
Developments in radiotherapy techniques, such as conformal radiotherapy, have increased the precision of radiotherapy and allowed dose escalation. Treatment is often combined with androgen deprivation therapy.

Brachytherapy
Brachytherapy involves the implantation of permanent radioactive seeds into the prostate. It offers a number of potential advantages over radical prostatectomy and external beam radiotherapy but is limited to patients at low risk with small glands (<50 cm^3).

Most patients report a worsening of lower urinary tract symptoms after brachytherapy, and about 5% will develop urinary retention. This technique therefore is not suitable for patients with significant lower urinary tract symptoms at presentation. Furthermore, if transurethral resection of the prostate is needed after brachytherapy, it may be very difficult and also is more likely to lead to postoperative incontinence.

High intensity focused ultrasound and cryotherapy
These two treatments are mentioned for completeness but are still largely experimental. High intensity focused ultrasound is undergoing clinical trials in the United Kingdom, and further data on safety and efficacy are awaited. Cryotherapy is available in some urological departments for the treatment of localised prostate cancer. Details on this technique are available through the further reading.

Hormone therapy
In most men with a life expectancy of more than 10 years, this option is unlikely to be appropriate. Treatment with hormones puts off the day when definitive treatment is required, while adding considerably to the morbidity. This option therefore is most appropriate for men with a life expectancy less than 10 years or when this is the patient's preference.

Locally advanced prostate cancer

In general, the treatment of patients in this category (stage T3 or T4 but without evidence of distant metastases) is with radiotherapy or hormones, or both. Active surveillance also is an option in older men and those with significant comorbidity and reduced life expectancy.

Management options for localised prostate cancer (stage T1 or T2)
- Active surveillance
- Radical prostatectomy
- External beam radiotherapy
- Brachytherapy
- High intensity focused ultrasound
- Cryotherapy
- Hormones

Active surveillance versus radical prostatectomy

A recent study that compared active surveillance with radical prostatectomy showed—after 10 years of follow up—a reduction in distant metastases, local progression, cancer specific death, and overall mortality in patients who underwent radical prostatectomy. Active surveillance thus perhaps is suited best to patients whose life expectancy is reduced for other reasons

---

Complications of external beam radiotherapy
- The incidence of long term erectile dysfunction after external beam radiotherapy is similar to that with radical prostatectomy but does not occur immediately
- Incontinence after radiotherapy occurs less commonly than with radical prostatectomy
- Bowel dysfunction (bleeding, passing mucus, and frequent bowel action) is a common acute complication of external beam radiotherapy and may become chronic in about 5% of cases

---

Potential advantages of brachytherapy over radical prostatectomy or external beam radiotherapy
- Usually performed as a day case procedure
- Risk of long term incontinence is low (about 1%)
- Erectile dysfunction may be preserved in the long term, although some studies show that up to 50% of patients potent before brachytherapy may develop erectile dysfunction over five years

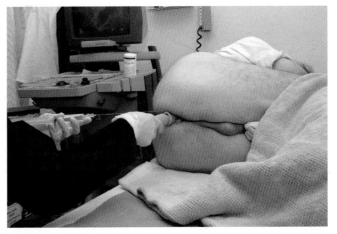

Ultrasound prostate biopsy—active surveillance is an option in elderly men with advanced prostate cancer. Some strategies for active surveillance include repeat biopsies every two years if radical treatments are suitable. With permission from Dr P Marazzi/Science Photo Library

Metastatic prostate cancer

Patients with metastatic prostate cancer cannot be cured. The emphasis of treatment is to control the extent and activity of the tumour by suppressing the levels of testosterone to castrate levels or by using androgen receptor blocking agents.

In patients with asymptomatic, small volume, bony metastases, active surveillance is an option, but complications related to the cancer, such as urinary obstruction and bone fractures, are reduced in patients who take hormone therapy. Patients with advanced metastases, particularly those at risk of spinal cord compression, should be offered immediate hormone therapy.

Customarily, an antiandrogen, such as cyproterone acetate, is prescribed for one week before and three weeks after the first dose of luteinising hormone releasing hormone analogue to prevent a transient stimulation of tumour growth. Luteinising hormone releasing hormone agonists act by initially stimulating luteinising hormone releasing hormone, so they produce a surge of testosterone. The latter may lead to spinal cord compression by bone metastases or urinary retention.

In most cases, the development of hormone resistant clones of cancer cells means that the prostate cancer will eventually become resistant to first line therapy. This will be apparent from successive rises in the levels of prostate specific antigen and, in some cases, the development of new bone metastases on the isotope bone scan.

Second line therapy can be given by the addition of an antiandrogen such as bicalutamide. Third and fourth line therapies are available, but most patients in this category will succumb to their disease. Palliative chemotherapy may be considered for hormone refractory disease.

Recent guidelines suggest that patients with prostate cancer that is metastatic and resistant to hormone treatment, even if asymptomatic, benefit from treatment with a bisphosphonate, such as zoledronic acid, to reduce the risk from, and time to development of, events such as bone pain, fracture, and spinal cord compression. Radiotherapy and strontium provide effective pain relief for bony metastatic disease.

Palliative care

In the terminal phases of metastatic prostate cancer, the patient and his carers recognise that the disease is progressing despite treatment and that the patient is reaching the end of his life. The focus in this phase moves towards quality of life and palliation of symptoms where appropriate. The involvement of an oncology nurse specialist and particularly a local palliative care team at this stage is invaluable.

The pictures of Gleason 3 and 5 prostate cancers were kindly supplied by Dr E Astall, consultant histopathologist, Peterborough and Stamford Hospitals Foundation Trust.

Symptoms and signs of spinal cord compression
- May present *de novo*
- Can present with numbness or paraesthesiae, "off legs," "falls," or "urinary difficulty"
- Prevention is better than cure—once lost, function is rarely regained

---

Management of spinal cord compression
- Admit for bed rest
- High doses of prednisolone
- Urgent magnetic resonance imaging of spine
- Admission to radiotherapy centre for radiotherapy
- Start hormone therapy with antiandrogen if patient is not already on hormone therapy

---

Recent advances

Laparoscopy
- Laparoscopic radical prostatectomy has been performed since 1997
- The procedure has a steep learning curve
- The procedure seems to have results similar to those with open radical prostatectomy (functional results and cancer control) but with faster convalescence and quicker return to normal activity

Robotics
- Robotic radical prostatectomy (for example, with the da Vinci system) provides greater manual dexterity than is possible with standard laparoscopic approaches
- The operator performs the procedure from a console and looks through binoculars at three dimensional view of the operative field
- Movement of the handles at the consoles determines the movement of laparoscopic instruments placed within the pelvis
- This procedure is said to be easier to learn than the standard laparoscopic procedure

Proteomics
- Proteomics is the study of protein expression and protein interactions
- Further study in this area may provide new markers for early detection of prostate cancer, assessment of the cancer's aggressiveness, monitoring after treatment, or predicting outcome after treatment

---

References
- Melia J. The burden of prostate cancer, its natural history, information on the outcome of screening and estimates of ad hoc screening with particular references to England and Wales. *BJU International* 2005;93(Suppl 3);4–15.
- Dawson C. Is radiological imaging worthwhile in patients with clinically localised prostate cancer? In: Dawson C, Muir G, eds. *The evidence for urology.* Harley: TfM Publishing, 2005.
- Bill-Axelson A, Holmberg L, Ruutu M, Haggman M, Andersson S-O, Bratell S, et al. Radical prostatectomy versus watchful waiting in early prostate cancer. *N Engl J Med* 2005;352:1977–84
- Scattoni V, Montorsi F, Picchio M, Roscigno M, Salonia A, Rigatti P, et al. Diagnosis of local recurrence after radical prostatectomy. *BJU International* 2004;93:680–8.
- Rees J, Patel B, Macdonagh R, Persad R. Cryosurgery for prostate cancer. *BJU International* 2004;93, 710–4.

8 Bladder cancer

Derek Fawcett

Aetiology

In the western world, bladder cancer is commonly a neoplasm of the transitional cells that line the urinary tract (transitional cell cancers). It is predominantly environmental in origin, being caused by carcinogens excreted in the urine. Bladder cancer is more common in men than women (3:1).

Workers in some occupations have an acknowledged risk of bladder cancer—for example, those in the rubber industry and those who handle aniline dyes. Industrially related cases of bladder cancer are decreasing now that regulations are in force to prevent the use of known carcinogens.

Specific aromatic amines (such as 2-naphthylamine and nitrosamines) are highly carcinogenic for the bladder and have been identified in cigarette smoke. Sadly, evidence supports the idea that many bladder cancers are related to cigarette smoking and are thus self-induced. Doctors in primary care have an important role in communicating the message that smoking causes cancers of the bladder, as well as other organs.

On a daily basis, we breathe many other environmental carcinogens that may also predispose to the development of bladder cancer.

Symptoms and signs of bladder cancer

Haematuria—the cardinal sign of bladder cancer—is classically painless and commonly is intermittent. All patients with macroscopic haematuria should be referred for investigation. An exception can be made in young women with a proved urinary tract infection, but these patients should also be referred for investigation if the haematuria persists despite treatment of the infection.

Macroscopic haematuria has a risk of 20–25% of cancer (bladder, renal, and prostatic) and the risk of detecting similar cancers in patients with microscopic haematuria is around 4%. Occasionally, bladder cancer presents with infection or is found incidentally on ultrasound. Investigation of microscopic haematuria is controversial, but currently the recommendation is that persistent evidence of haematuria on microscopy or dipstick testing in patients older than 40 years should be referred for investigation.

Primary carcinoma in situ rarely presents with haematuria. It may present with irritative symptoms.

Investigation of patients with suspected bladder cancer

All patients with bladder cancer should be managed by urologists who are part of a multidisciplinary team associated with a cancer network.

Initial investigations
Most patients now are seen in specialist haematuria clinics. Fibre optic cystoscopy under local anaesthetic will be the initial investigation. This may show a classic papillary tumour (fronded and like seaweed) or a tumour that is more broad based (sessile) and less papillary and solid looking, which may be invasive.

> **Adenomacarcinoma and squamous cell carcinoma**
> - In areas of endemic schistosomiasis (caused by *Schistosoma haematobium*), most bladder cancers are squamous cell cancers, although this parasitic infection may produce transitional cell cancer
> - Squamous cancers also may occur in older women with chronic urinary tract infection and may present in bladder diverticulae
> - Adenocarcinoma of the bladder classically arises in a urachal remnant, from areas of metaplasia, or from direct invasion from the colon
> - The bladder is also the site of rarer tumours, including phaeochromocytomas and rhabdomyosarcomas (in children)
> - If bladder adenocarcinoma is detected, a primary site outside the bladder should be excluded before assuming a primary bladder origin

> **Important signs and symptoms**
> - Macroscopic haematuria never must be ignored
> - Patients with macroscopic haematuria must be referred at the time of first presentation
> - Recurrent microscopic or dipstick haematuria in patients of either sex older than 40 years should be referred

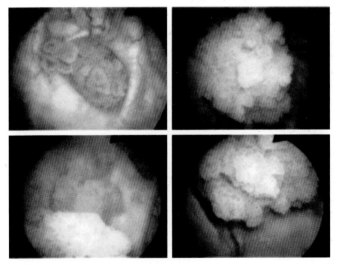

Papillary transitional cell carcinoma

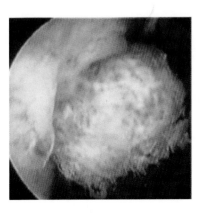

Sessile transitional cell carcinoma

29

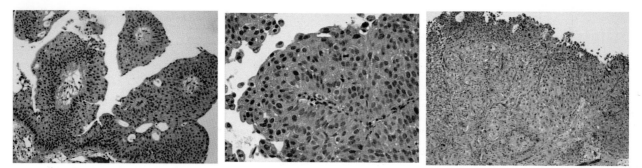

Transitional cell cancer stages: G1—well differentiated (left), G2—moderately differentiated (centre), and G3—poorly differentiated (right)

Specimens of urine will be taken for culture and cytology, and imaging of the urinary tract will be arranged. Cytology of the urine may be affected by the instrumentation of the urinary tract, so samples for cytology should be sent before the cystoscopy is performed.

Imaging

Some debate remains about the ideal imaging method for patients with haematuria and suspected bladder cancer. Traditionally, the intravenous pyelogram is the standard, but it must be complemented with ultrasound to exclude mass lesions of the kidney. Ultrasound alone is almost certainly inadequate. Cross sectional imaging (computed tomography or magnetic resonance imaging) is reserved for staging muscle invasive bladder cancer.

Definitive diagnosis

The definitive diagnosis is made on biopsy, which is commonly taken with a rigid cystoscope or resectoscope under anaesthesia. Bladder muscle must be included in the biopsy to exclude or confirm muscle invasion—the single most important prognostic feature of bladder cancer.

Bimanual examination under anaesthesia is essential in the assessment of bladder cancer, as the clinical stage or category will become apparent. A palpable mass after resection is a good guide to arranging computed tomography or magnetic resonance imaging before the results of biopsies are known.

Histological types and grading

Transitional cell and squamous cell cancers of the bladder are described by histopathologists in three grades: G1 (well differentiated, G2 (moderately differentiated), and G3 (poorly differentiated). These grades represent the overall level of dedifferentiation from normal histology and architecture. They have prognostic value and different treatment pathways.

Staging

Clinical staging (T category) is established by bimanual examination at cystoscopy and biopsy under anaesthetic. Pathological staging is determined by the histopathologist after examination of the biopsy. It is denoted by the prefix "p." Biopsies can be staged only up to stage pT2a, as staging higher than this requires a whole specimen from cystectomy.

Treatment of bladder cancer

Superficial bladder cancer (pTa and pT1)

The overall aim of treatment in superficial bladder cancer (pTa and pT1) is preservation of the bladder and achievement of a normal life expectancy by detecting progression and preventing recurrence. This is achieved in most cases by a combination of treatment and surveillance (check or review cystoscopy).

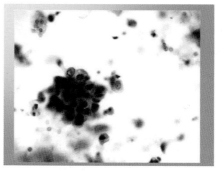

Cytology of voided urine showing a clump of malignant cells

Clinical staging

Stage	Description
T1	Impalpable before and after resection
T2	Palpable before but not after resection
T3	Palpable before and after resection
T4	Involving a neighbouring organ

Pathological staging

Stage	Description	Bladder cancer
PTa	Confined to urothelium; basement membrane not breached	Superficial
pT1	Invasion into lamina propria	Superficial (invasive)
PTis	Overtly malignant cells form a layer that replaces urothelium	
pT2a	Invasion into muscularis propria (detrusor)	Muscle invasive
pT2b	Deep invasion into muscularis propria (detrusor)	Muscle invasive
pT3a	Microscopic extravesical spread	Muscle invasive
pT3b	Macroscopic extravesical spread	Muscle invasive
pT4	Involves neighbouring organ	

Involved lymph nodes

Nodal disease indicates a very poor prognosis. The TNM classification classifies it as follows:
- N1: single node <2 cm
- N2: single node >2 cm, multiple nodes <5 cm
- N3: >5 cm

Metastases

The TNM classification classifies soft tissue or bony metastases as follows:
- M1: presence of metastases

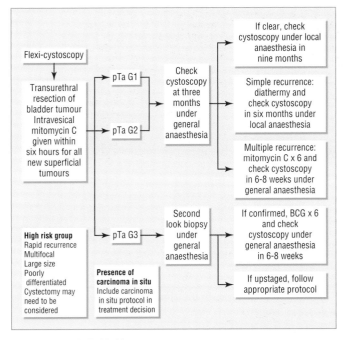

Management of pTa bladder cancer

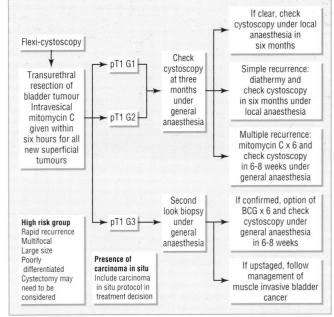

Management of pT1 bladder cancer

Newly diagnosed superficial bladder cancer is resected under general anaesthesia (transurethral resection of bladder tumour). A single instillation of mitomycin C is given into the bladder within 6–24 hours of resection. In patients with superficial bladder cancer, the instillation of mitomycin C within a few hours of resection significantly reduces the incidence of recurrent disease at three months.

The use of intravesical BCG as a non-specific immune stimulant is now standard practice in patients with high grade superficial bladder cancer (pTa G3, pT1 G3, or pTis). It is given in a course of weekly instillations for six weeks.

Symptoms severe enough to require antituberculous treatment can occur in up to 6% of patients. Systemic infection with BCG has been responsible for several deaths.

It must be recognised that pT1 disease is already showing invasive potential and has a significant risk of progression. The overall intention of treatment is preservation of the bladder and achievement of normal life expectancy.

Poorly differentiated tumours (pT1 G3) are always subject to repeat biopsy to confirm the stage. If confirmed, intravesical immunotherapy is indicated (six instillations of BCG). If muscle invasion is detected, the protocol for pT2 tumours is followed.

Widespread pT1 G3 tumour associated with carcinoma in situ is a dangerous situation, and serious consideration should be given to early radical cystectomy. Cross sectional imaging should be performed before radical surgery is considered.

Carcinoma in situ

Although classified as superficial bladder cancer, carcinoma in situ is a completely different type of disorder that carries a high risk of progression to muscle invasive, and hence life threatening, bladder cancer. The prime intention of treatment is to eradicate the changes by immunotherapy, maintain surveillance, and predict and prevent progression to cystectomy.

Carcinoma in situ of the urinary bladder (pTis) is traditionally included under the heading of superficial bladder cancer, because it is superficial and the basement membrane is not breached. It is at the end of the spectrum of dysplasia of the urothelium. The cells, however, cytologically are malignant, and the tumour may progress rapidly to muscle invasive cancer.

Common side effects of treatment with BCG instillation

- Bladder irritability:
  Dysuria
  Frequency
  Haematuria
- Fever
- Malaise
- Nausea
- Chills
- Arthralgia
- Pruritus
- Granulomatous prostatitis

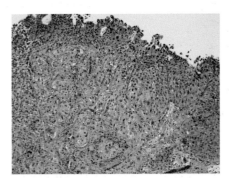

pT1 G3 bladder tumour

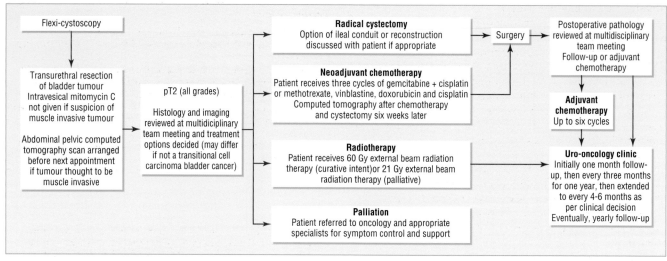

Management of muscle invasive bladder cancer

Traditionally, BCG is given in weekly instillations for six weeks followed by a check cystoscopy and biopsy at three months. Debate remains as to whether BCG prevents progression of carcinoma in situ to invasive bladder cancer.

Widespread primary carcinoma in situ is very dangerous, and serious consideration should be given to early radical cystectomy, instead of attempting to conserve the bladder by the use of BCG. Rarely, carcinoma in situ may metastasise without an apparent "tumour" in the bladder.

Muscle invasive bladder cancer (pT2 and pT3)
Muscle invasive bladder cancer is a life threatening disease that requires meticulous staging and treatment planning. In patients with reasonable life expectancy and localised disease, the intention of treatment is cure, but in elderly people, palliation may be a preferable strategy.

Primary surgery
Primary surgery is the treatment of choice if the patient is fit. In men, surgery comprises cystoprostatectomy and pelvic node dissection, but in women it needs anterior pelvic clearance, with a hysterectomy, salpingo-oophorectomy, and upper third vaginectomy. Mortality should be <2%. Such surgery should be carried out only in centres that perform large amounts routinely. In patients unfit for surgery or who prefer to avoid surgery, external beam radiotherapy is an alternative.

Neoadjuvant and adjuvant chemotherapy
The role of neoadjuvant chemotherapy remains uncertain, but downstaging achieved with neoadjuvant chemotherapy seems to lead to a better outcome. Adjuvant chemotherapy has little evidence in its favour and is of doubtful value.

Urinary diversion after bladder removal
Bladder removal is followed by a cutaneous diversion (ileal conduit) or by orthotopic or ectopic bladder reconstruction (neobladder). In the early 1950s, Bricker introduced the concept of interposing a section of small bowel between the ureters and skin as a conduit (ileal conduit). This allowed the construction of a larger and non-stenosing stoma over which a bag could be fitted. The ileal conduit has remained the mainstay of urinary diversion after cystectomy ever since. Efforts to create a replacement urinary reservoir have led to the creation of orthotopic reservoirs that are attached to the native urethra, thus allowing urine to be expressed in the normal way.

Complications of urinary division
- Electrolyte and acid-base balance
  Hyperchloraemic metabolic acidosis
  Can lead to electrolyte abnormalities, osteomalacia, altered liver metabolism, renal stones, and abnormal drug metabolism
- Deterioration in renal function—may result, for example, from chronic retention or infection in neobladders or stenosis of uretero-ileal junction in an ileal conduit.
- Bone disease—from chronic acidosis
- Impairment of growth and development (in children)
- Mucus production in intestinal segments used in diversion or reconstruction
- Infection
- Development of stones
- Rupture (in orthotopic neobladders)
- Tumour formation—exact risk of development of adenocarcinoma in intestinal segment used for reconstruction or diversion unknown

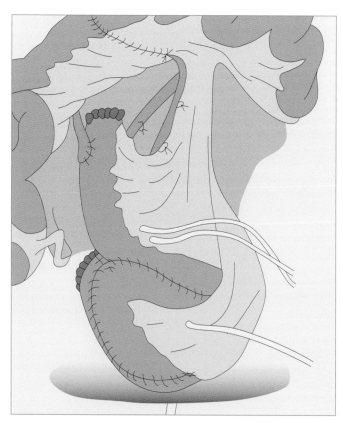

"Studer" type orthotopic neobladder

Palliative care in bladder cancer

If death from bladder cancer is inevitable, priority must be given to preventing death from locally recurrent disease and the associated misery of bleeding and strangury.

The old surgeon's prayer "Pray it not be my tongue or my bladder" is indicative of the misery that bladder cancer causes in its late stages. Pain, bleeding, strangury, and fistulation are typical end stage problems in all types of pelvic cancer. In the presence of incurable disease, various methods can be used to reduce the incidence of these symptoms.

A team approach—with urologist, clinical oncologist, palliative care doctor, clinical nurse specialists, and pain control team—should provide a multidisciplinary approach to palliation. This requires use of good symptom relief with pain control, palliative radiotherapy, or palliative chemotherapy: all of which aim to improve the quality of life and reduce pain and bleeding.

Urinary diversion or even cystectomy are justified as palliative measures for bleeding, pain, and fistulation. Good practice is to consider the possible consequences of late local recurrence when deciding the initial treatment strategies at presentation.

Bladder cancer (new or end stage) that presents with bilateral ureteric obstruction and acute renal failure is particularly difficult to manage for the admitting team. Nephrostomies can be easily inserted to prevent immediate death, but patients rarely survive more than a few weeks and allowing death at presentation occasionally may be an appropriate decision.

Further reading

- Oosterlink W, Lobel B, Jakse G, Malmström P-U, Stöckle M, Sternberg C, et al. Guidelines on bladder cancer. *Eur Urol* 2002; 41:105–12.
- Gerharz EW, Turner WH, Kalble T, Woodhouse CRJ. Metabolic and functional consequences of urinary reconstruction with bowel. *BJU International* 2003;91:143–9.
- Meyer J-P, Fawcett D, Gillatt D, Persad R. Orthotopic neobladder reconstruction—what are the options? *BJU International* 2005; 96:493–7.
- Studer UE, Varol C, Danuser H. Surgical atlas—orthotopic ileal neobladder. *Br J Urol* 2004: 93; 183–93.

I thank Nicky Sillwood Clinical Nurse Specialist in Uro-Oncology, Harold Hopkins Department of Urology, Royal Berkshire Hospital, and Natalie Scott-Young, special reader in histopathology, Royal Berkshire Hospital, Reading. The line drawing of the Studer type orthotopic neobladder is adapted from Studer UE, et al. *BJU Int* 2004;93:183–93. With permission of the publishers, Blackwell Publishing.

9 Renal and testis cancer

Paul K Hegarty

Renal cancer

Presentation

The classic triad of flank pain, haematuria, and palpable mass thankfully now is rare. Such a presentation usually denotes a locally advanced cancer. A paraneoplasia is found in 20% of cases, which is why renal cell carcinoma previously was known as the "physician's disease."

Investigation

Diagnosis of renal cell carcinoma begins with a full history and examination. Although most varicoceles arise in the absence of any other condition, a newly developed varicocoele on the left side in the presence of a left renal tumour implies renal vein involvement, usually at a stage where the primary tumour is palpable. A full blood count; erythrocyte sedimentation rate; and serum calcium, liver, and renal profiles all are indicated to exclude any of the associated paraneoplastic conditions.

Imaging

The diagnosis of renal cell carcinoma is largely radiological, with biopsy seldom used. Ultrasonography allows diagnosis of many renal tumours nowadays and is particularly good at distinguishing solid masses from simple cysts. Ultrasound also provides good imaging to determine involvement of the inferior vena cava. Staging of renal cell carcinoma is primarily by high quality abdominal computed tomography. A chest x ray is usually sufficient to stage the thorax. Magnetic resonance imaging can be used when venous involvement is suspected or the patient is allergic to intravenous contrast medium. Three dimensional computer reconstruction of computed tomography or magnetic resonance imaging is essential for planning surgery nephron-sparing surgery.

Genetics

Knudson and Strong proposed that a gene product that could suppress tumour development must be involved in carcinogenesis. They suggested that mutation or inactivation of both alleles of this "tumour suppressor gene" would be needed for the evolution of cancer. They thus proposed a "two hit" theory of carcinogenesis. Their hypothesis has been proved for a number of cancers, including renal cell carcinoma. Von Hippel-Lindau disease is an autosomal dominant disorder that occurs in one per 36 000 population. Half of such cases develop renal cell carcinoma.

The gene for Von Hippel-Lindau disease is a tumour suppressor gene on chromosome 3. It contains three exons and encodes a protein of 213 amino acids. Loss of its activity favours tumour growth. Abnormalities in the gene for Von Hippel-Lindau disease are evident in 75% of sporadic cases of renal cell carcinoma. Furthermore, mutation of p53 has been reported in 6-40% of cases of renal cell carcinoma and may correlate with tumour grade and stage.

Features of Von Hippel-Lindau disease

- Phaeochromocytoma
- Retinal angiomata
- Hemangioblastomas of the brain stem, cerebellum, or spinal cord
- Renal cysts
- Pancreatic cysts and adenocarcinoma
- Epididymal cystadenoma
- Endolymphatic sac tumour in ear (<0.5%)

> **Paraneoplasia is a clinical or biochemical disturbance associated with malignant tumours not related directly to invasion by the primary tumour or metastasis**

Rank order of paraneoplastic processes in renal cell carcinoma

Process	Patients affected(%)
Raised erythrocyte sedimentation rate	55.0
Hypertension	37.0
Anaemia	36.0
Weight loss	34.0
Pyrexia	17.0
Abnormal results of liver function test	14.0
Raised levels of serum calcium	5.0
Raised levels of haemoglobin	3.5
Neuromyopathy	3.2
Amyloidosis	2.0

Stauffer's syndrome: abnormal liver function test and raised prothrombin time

---

TNM classification of renal cancer (1997)

Stage	Definition
T1	<7 cm confined to kidney
T2	>7 cm confined to kidney
T3a	Into adrenal or perinephric fat not Gerota's fascia
T3b	Involvement of the vena cava below diaphragm
T3c	Involvement of the vena cava above diaphragm
T4	Beyond Gerota's fascia
N1	One regional node
N2	More than one regional node
M1	Distant metastases

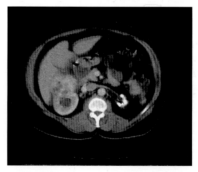

Computed tomogram of the abdomen with intravenous contrast demonstrating tumour arising from right kidney and tiny left kidney

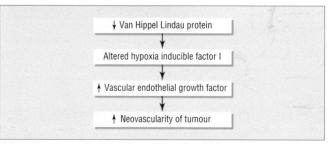

Proposed pathway of effect of loss of Von Hippel-Lindau gene activity

Treatment

Observation

The growth rate and risk of metastasis of small renal tumours (<3 cm diameter) that are discovered incidentally are low. They may be managed by observation in unfit patients or those with short life expectancy.

Surgery

Removal of all of the tumour currently offers the best chance of cure. Traditionally, open radical nephrectomy was indicated for all cases without metastasis. Partial nephrectomy allows preservation of ipsilateral renal function.

Open nephrectomy remains necessary for large primary tumours or those with involvement of the inferior vena cava. Nephrectomy may also be performed to "debulk" the tumour load before immunotherapy with interferon.

Ablation

Small cancers may be treated by cryotherapy or radiofrequency ablation. These tumours need to be imaged clearly and are targeted best if they are on the periphery of the kidney. These methods hold great promise but must be proved to match standard surgery in oncological control.

Adjuvant therapy

Chemotherapy—Renal cell cancer is resistant to chemotherapy. Renal cancer cells express transmembrane proteins that actively pump out large hydrophobic compounds, including several of the cytotoxic drugs.

Immonotherapy—Various immunotherapeutic regimens have been described, with combined complete and partial responses at best of up to 30%. Interferon alpha and, more commonly, interleukin 2 are used to treat metastatic disease, especially after debulking of the primary tumour with surgery. Patients who may be amenable to immunotherapy tend to have non-bulky pulmonary or soft tissue metastases, or both. Patients with bony metastases respond poorly to immunotherapy.

Radiotherapy—Radiation is used for symptomatic bone or brain metastases.

Testis cancer

Cancer of the testis is the commonest cancer occuring in men aged between 15 and 35 years. The lifetime risk is one in 500.

High rates of cure in patients with testis cancer are the result of modern multidisciplinary treatments. They are unrivalled in patients with other solid tumours. These enviable results are dependent on the doctor and rely on a team approach that combines urological surgery, chemotherapy, and radiotherapy.

Early presentation is the patient factor that determines cure rates. Symptomatic delay has a proved negative impact on disease stage, treatment outcome, and mortality.

Presentation

Most cases of testis cancer present with a scrotal mass or discomfort. Advanced cases can present with back pain, respiratory compromise, or neurological deficit. Examination should not be restricted to the scrotum; it should include the abdomen and supraclavicular fossa.

Markers

Alpha fetoprotein is raised in embryonal carcinoma, teratocarcinoma, yolk sac tumour, or combined tumours but not with pure choriocarcinoma or pure seminoma. Human chorionic

---

> **Innovation in laparoscopy allows total and partial nephrectomy to be informed with minimal invasion**

Partial nephrectomy

- Used to be reserved for patients with bilateral tumours, solitary kidney tumours, and current or possible future renal impairment
- Increasingly offered to patients with normal contralateral renal function

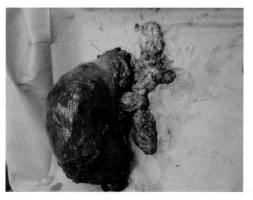

Right radical nephrectomy specimen. Note the adrenal gland superomedially and tumour extension into the inferior vena cava and contralateral vein

Classification of testis cancer

Germ cell tumours

- Seminoma (35%)
- Non-seminomatous germ cell tumours

Non-germ cell tumours (5–6%)

- Leydig cell tumours
- Sertoli cell tumours (very rare)
- Lymphoma (secondary tumour)

Non-seminomatous germ cell tumour

- Non-seminomatous germ cell tumour occurs typically in men aged 20–35 years
- Histological types comprise embryonal carcinoma, teratoma, choriocarcinoma, and yolk sac elements alone or mixed
- More aggressive and less chemosensitive and radiosensitive than seminoma
- In the presence of seminoma and non-seminomatous elements, the clinical behaviour is regarded as non-seminomatous germ cell tumour.

Seminoma

- Classic seminoma occurs typically in men in their 30s
- Relatively slow growing and chemosensitive and radiosensitive
- Anaplastic type has greater mitotic activity, with higher rate of local invasion
- Spermatocytic type often occurs in men older than 50 years and has a low metastatic potential

Prognosis of testis cancer based on marker levels

Prognos	Proport (%)	Markers			Survial (%)
		AFP	Human chorionic gonadotrophin (IU)	Lactate dehydrogenase (×normal)	
Good	56	AFP	<1 000	<1.5	90
Intermedi	28	AFP	1 000–10 000	1.5–10	80
Poor	16	AFP	>10 000	>10	50

gonadotrophin is raised in all patients with choriocarcinoma, 40–60% with embryonal carcinoma, and 5–10% with pure seminoma (apparently produced by the syncytiotrophoblast-like giant cells that occur in some seminomas). Lactate dehydrogenase is found in seminomas and non-seminomatous germ cell tumours in proportion to the disease stage. Placental alkaline phosphate is a fetal isoenzyme; its levels are raised in 40% of patients with advanced seminoma.

Levels of markers before treatment correlate with prognosis. Normalisation of levels of markers after treatment cannot be equated with the absence of residual disease. Between 10% and 20% of patients who receive combined systemic chemotherapy for bulky metastatic disease and subsequently undergo retroperitoneal dissection of the lymph nodes have a histologically confirmed viable tumour despite having normal preoperative levels of markers.

Staging
The Royal Marsden Hospital's system of staging requires cross sectional imaging of the abdomen, usually with computed tomography. If the abdomen is involved, imaging should include the thorax, otherwise a plain chest x ray will suffice.

Treatment
Initial treatment is urgent radical orchidectomy. This is performed through an inguinal incision. The testis and cord are delivered and isolated from the wound. The spermatic cord is ligated at the deep ring. A non-absorbable suture facilitates future identification in the event of retroperitoneal dissection of the lymph nodes being indicated. If the diagnosis is in doubt, the spermatic cord is placed in a soft clamp before the isolated testis is bivalved.

Sperm bank facilities should be made available before the operation. Orchidectomy allows tissue diagnosis to guide further treatment if necessary. In stage I seminoma, the primary tumour's size is an independent risk factor for subsequent relapse. Negative prognostic factors include presence of lymphatic or vascular invasion. In non-seminomatous germ cell tumours, the absence of yolk sac elements or the presence of embryonal cell carcinoma worsens prognosis.

Abdominal computed tomography can be performed before or after surgery. Patients who present with symptomatic extralymphatic metastases (stage IV) may need emergency chemotherapy, with orchidectomy deferred until their overall status has improved.

Subsequent management depends on the type and stage of the tumour. Retroperitoneal dissection of the lymph nodes virtually removes the chance of relapse in the abdomen. About 25% of patients with clinical stage I non-seminomatous germ cell tumours have microscopic retroperitoneal lymph node involvement. Men with this clinical diagnosis can be offered primary retroperitoneal dissection of the lymph nodes, chemotherapy, or close surveillance of markers and imaging. Treatment of residual mass on imaging after chemotherapy is controversial and requires multidisciplinary input. The main complications of retroperitoneal lymph node dissection are loss of anterograde ejaculation and lymphocoele formation. Recent advances in laparoscopic surgery are exploring its application to this retroperitoneal operation.

Royal Marsden Hospital's staging system

Stage	Description
I	Tumour confined to testis
IIA	Regional nodes <2 cm
IIB	Regional nodes 2–5 cm
IIC	Regional nodes >5 cm
III	Supradiaphragmatic lymphadenopathy
IV	Extralymphatic involvement

TNM classification of testis tumours (1997)

Stage	Description
T0	No evidence of primary tumour
Tis	Carcinoma in situ
T1	Tumour limited to testis and epididymis without vascular or lymphatic invasion
T2	Tumour limited to testis and epididymis with vascular or lymphatic invasion, or tumour extending through tunica albuginea with involvement of tunica vaginalis
T3	Tumour invades spermatic cord
T4	Tumour invades scrotum
N0	No regional lymph node metastasis
N1	Metastasis with a lymph node mass ≤2 cm and five or fewer positive nodes
N2	Metastasis with a lymph node mass >2 cm but <5 cm in diameter, or more than five positive nodes
N3	Metastasis with a lymph node mass >5 cm in greatest dimension

Treatment according to tumour type and stage

Stage	Seminoma	Non-seminomatous germ cell tumour
I	Orchidectomy ± irradiation or chemotherapy or surveillance	Orchidectomy ±retroperitoneal dissection of the lymph nodes or surveillance
IIa and IIb	Orchidectomy + chemotherapy	Orchidectomy+chemotherapy or retroperitoneal dissection of the lymph nodes
IIc and III	Orchidectomy + chemotherapy	Orchidectomy+ chemotherapy
IV	Chemotherapy ± orchidectomy	Chemotherapy ± orchidectomy

Further reading
- Walsh PC, Retik AB. *Campbell's urology*. Philadelphia, PA: Saunders, 2002.
- Chisholm GD. Nephrogenic ridge tumors and their syndrome. *Ann N Y Acad Sci* 1874;230;403–23.
- Knudson AG, Strong LC. Mutation and cancer: a model for Wilm's tumor of the kidney. *J Natl Cancer Inst* 1972;48:313–24.

10 Urinary tract stone disease

Hugh N Whitfield

Prevalence

Ten per cent of the population in the United Kingdom may expect to have an episode of stone disease during their lifetime. The upper urinary tract is affected in most cases.

Bladder stones are found in a small proportion of men with bladder outflow obstruction. The incidence in children remains high in some developing countries.

The prevalence of renal stones varies; it also correlates with affluence. A "stone belt" can be traced across India, Pakistan, and North America. The prevalence of stones changes with age and is lower in women, although the male:female ratio is becoming more equal.

Presentation

Renal stones
Renal stones may be suspected because of loin pain. The most severe pain occurs when stones are moving. Paradoxically, therefore, large stones that are in the kidney and not moving may cause less discomfort than smaller stones that are moving. In some patients, pain is provoked by exercise. Asymptomatic stones often are found during radiographic or ultrasound imaging for unrelated reasons.

Ureteric stones
When stones are moving out of the kidney into and down the ureter, the acute colicky pain is second to none in its severity. When a ureteric stone has been present for ≥72 hours, the acute pain subsides and the patient has relatively few symptoms. Chronic ureteric obstruction is dangerous, because the lack of symptoms may lull the patient (and an ill informed medical adviser) into a false sense of security. A stone that is lodged in the intramural ureter causes strangury and discomfort that is felt at the tip of the penis in men.

Investigation

Renal stones
However renal stones are diagnosed initially, treatment can be planned only after an intravenous urogram, which enables the relation of the stone to the pelvicaliceal system to be identified. The management of large or bilateral renal stones, or both, depends on the patient's overall and differential renal function.

Glomerular filtration rate is measured most accurately by an isotopic plasma clearance method with the use of ethylenediaminetetraacetic acid (EDTA). Differential renal function can be assessed by static or dynamic renograms with dimercaptosuccinic acid (DMSA) or mercaptoacetylglycine (MAGIII), respectively.

Ureteric stones
Debate continues about the best imaging method to be used in patients who present with suspected acute renal or ureteric colic. Intravenous urography and computed tomography have their own advantages and disadvantages. Conservative expectant management of a ureteric stone thought to be small enough to pass spontaneously can only be pursued safely if the patient is monitored with the use of renographic methods.

Differential diagnosis of ureteric colic

- Appendicitis
- Diverticulitis
- Salpingitis
- Pyelonephritis
- Leaking aortic aneurysm

Absence of pain does not indicate absence of chronic obstruction, which can cause irreversible renal damage

---

Advantages of intravenous urography over computed tomography

- More readily available
- Less irradiation
- Easy to interpret
- More economical
- Shows ureteric anatomy better

Advantages of computed tomography over intravenous urography

- Quick
- No risk of contrast allergy
- High specificity
- Shows other pathology
- Not contraindicated in patients with diabetes who are taking metformin

---

Percentage of ureteric stones that pass spontaneously

Size of stone (mm)	Stones that pass spontaneously (%)
<4	90
4–6	50
>6	20

Treatment

Renal stones

Five options for the treatment of renal stones exist:

- *Conservative management*—Conservative management of small renal stones has been advocated. The only good randomised trial, however, has provided evidence to suggest that such stones are treated better with extracorporeal shockwave lithotripsy. Staghorn calculi also may be asymptomatic; conservative management has been shown to be contraindicated unless comorbidity is very considerable.
- *Extracorporeal shockwave lithotripsy*—This method is effective for treating kidney stones <2 cm in maximum diameter, as long as no obstruction to the passage of stone fragments is present. Ninety-nine per cent of patients can tolerate the procedure after no more than a non-steroidal anti-inflammatory drug. More than one treatment session may be needed in patients with large or hard stones. The larger the stone, the greater the risk that fragments will cause a blockage in the ureter that has to be relieved endoscopically.
- *Retrograde renoscopy*—A laser fibre can be introduced through a flexible fibre optic ureterorenoscope, which is introduced through the urethra and bladder, and up the ureter to the renal collecting system. Stones ≤1 cm in diameter can be disintegrated.
- *Percutaneous nephrolithotomy*—Stones >2 cm in diameter may be treated by percutaneous nephrolithotomy. Under fluoroscopic control, a track with a diameter of about 1 cm is dilated transparenchymally into the collecting system. Disintegrating devices, which can be introduced through a nephroscope, are used to break the stone into fragments that can be evacuated through the track.
- *Open surgery*—This is needed infrequently. Staghorn stones, in which the bulk of the stone lies within calices rather than within the renal pelvis, are treated best by open surgery. Kidneys that contribute <10% of overall renal function should usually be removed. Extensive perirenal fibrosis is usually encountered, which makes such a nephrectomy impossible laparoscopically.

Ureteric stones

Five options for the management of ureteric stones exist. The decision depends on the severity and length of time of the symptoms, the size and site of the stone, evidence of renal functional impairment, and, sometimes, on the patient's domestic or work plans.

- *Conservative management*—Most stones ≤5 mm in maximum diameter are likely to pass spontaneously and should be allowed to do so. Best practice, however, demands that conservative management is monitored renographically every two weeks. This is difficult to achieve. Patients often are advised to drink copious volumes of fluid to "flush the stone through." No evidence shows that this helps, and, for good reasons, this approach may be counterproductive. Stones will pass down the ureter when the ureter peristalses. In the presence of an obstruction, diuresis will provoke ureteric dilatation and reduce peristalsis. Anticholinergic drugs, such as hyosine, similarly will be ineffective.
- *Extracorporeal shockwave lithotripsy*—This has been advocated for ureteric stones, when imaging is possible radiographically or by ultrasound. This approach is less successful for ureteric stones than renal stones and is possible only at urological centres that have a static rather than mobile lithotripter.
- *Endoscopic ureterolithotomy*—With or without stone disintegration, this is a safe and effective method of managing ureteric stones that need intervention.

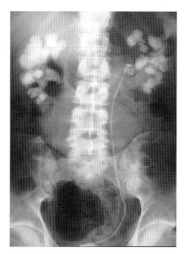

Bilateral staghorn calculi

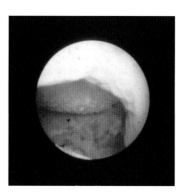

Percutaneous nephrolithotomy—view from a calyx of a stone in the renal pelvis

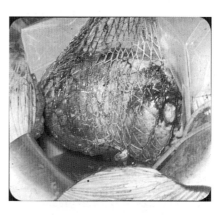

Open surgery

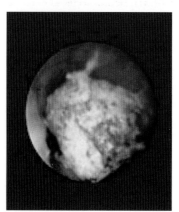

Stone in ureter

- *Open surgery*—This is indicated very rarely for ureteric stones. If associated ureteric pathology, such as stricture, is present, open surgery may be the only solution.
- *Laparoscopy*—Does not play any important role in the management of uteric stone disease.

Causes and prevention of renal stones

The need for metabolic screening in people who produce stones is controversial. Some people advocate screening only in people with recurrent stones. As 80% of people who produce their first stone will have a recurrence within 10 years, however, this distinction can be regarded as irrelevant. Patients who recently have experienced an episode of renal colic are well motivated to do whatever is possible to prevent another similar episode. Appropriate preventative measures can be recommended only when the results of metabolic screening for stones are available.

Analysis of the composition of a stone is a useful start. Serum levels of uric acid and corrected serum levels of calcium should be measured. Collection of urine for 24 hours is needed to measure excretion of calcium, oxalate, uric acid, and citrate.

Most stones are composed of calcium oxalate. Many predisposing factors exist: the most common is low intake of fluid. Patients who work in hot environments, those who take a lot of exercise, and people who fly long distances are at considerably increased risk. People who form stones should aim to have a urine output of two litres a day and need to drink enough to ensure this is achieved.

Idiopathic hypercalciuria is a frequent finding. If this persists despite appropriate dietary changes and fluid intake, treatment with a thiazide diuretic can be helpful.

Raised levels of uric acid in the blood or urine are important causes of stone formation. If a reduction in protein intake is not enough to correct the biochemistry, allopurinol should be given. Recurrence of stones composed of uric acid should be preventable, except in patients with an ileostomy, who have an increased risk of urate stones because of their acidic urine, which cannot be made more alkaline.

Urinary infection may cause large stones composed of triple (calcium, magnesium, and ammonium) phosphate, particularly in women with organisms that split urea. Recurrence of stones caused by infection can be prevented if the stone is removed completely and the urine is kept sterile.

Biochemical abnormalities in urine caused by excessive dietary intake of some foods or fluids can be treated effectively by dietary changes. Patients are often unaware of the dietary risk factors. Congenital causes of stones—for example, cystine—are uncommon. Advice from a nephrologist is needed.

Risk factors for people who form stones of calcium oxalate

- Male sex
- Low urinary volume
- Hyperoxaluria
- Increased urinary pH
- Hypercalciuria
- Hyperuricosuria
- Hypocitraturia
- Hypomagnesuria

General dietary advice for people who form stones of calcium oxalate

- Maintain urine volume of two litres a day
- Reduce intake of oxalate
- Aim for intake of calcium of 750 mg/day
- Consume no added salt
- Consume a diet high in fibre

Further reading

- Whitfield HN, W F Hendry WF, Kirby RS, Duckett JW (eds). *Textbook of genitourinary surgery*. Oxford: Blackwell Science, 1998.
- Whitfield HN. The management of ureteric stones. Part I: diagnosis. *BJU Int* 1999;84:8:911–5.
- Whitfield HN. The management of ureteric stones. Part II: therapy. *BJU Int* 1999;84:8:916–21.
- Whitfield HN. Stone disease. In: Gerharz EW, Emberton M, O'Brien T, (eds) *Classic papers in urology*. Oxford: Isis Medical Media, 2000; pp 295–315.

11 Common paediatric problems

A R Prem

Phimosis

Phimosis is the most common reason for circumcision, although recurrent balanitis is also an indication. Circumcision may also be performed for religious or social reasons.

At birth, adhesions are present between the glans penis and foreskin, but separation begins to occur immediately and continues thereafter. The prepuce normally becomes retractile after the age of two years, but many adolescent boys retain some adhesions. Preputial adhesions are a common reason for referral to a urologist, but adhesions are normal and should be treated only if "physiological phimosis" persists into adolescence and causes problems with masturbation or sexual intercourse. A non-retractile foreskin is free of symptoms and self-limiting, and circumcision is not needed. Parents often say that the prepuce "balloons" when the child urinates, but this is a sign of a non-retractile foreskin rather than phimosis. Careful examination will show that the urethral meatus is visible through the narrowed preputial opening, and, with time, this opening widens to allow the foreskin to retract normally. True or "pathologic phimosis" is rare, but it may cause appreciable problems in childhood or adolescence. Treatment usually is circumcision, although alternative treatments, such as preputioplasty or application of steroid creams, may be needed.

Undescended testis

The incidence of undescended testis ranges from 3.4% to 5.8% in full term boys but decreases to 0.8% in boys aged about one year. Why testes fail to descend into the scrotum is unclear, but recent evidence suggests that descent occurs in two distinct phases and that androgens may have an important role, possibly acting via the genitofemoral nerve. An undescended testis can be classified by its location in the upper scrotum, superficial inguinal pouch, inguinal canal, or abdomen. In 80% of cases, the undescended testis will be palpable in the inguinal canal. Patients with undescended testes have two major concerns: increased incidence of testicular cancer and heightened risk of subfertility.

For treatment purposes, the main distinction that needs to be made is whether the testis is palpable. If the testis is palpable in the inguinal canal, an orchidopexy should be carried out. The correct timing of orchidopexy has been debated. Spontaneous descent of undescended testis is rare after the age of one year.

Every attempt should be made to locate an impalpable testis. Ultrasound, computed tomography, and magnetic resonance imaging have been used, but laparoscopy is the current investigation of choice. If blind ending spermatic vessels are noted, further evaluation is not needed; the patient and parents should be counselled and hormonal replacement and a testicular prosthesis may be needed. If the testis is intra-abdominal in a prepubertal child, orchidopexy should be performed as soon as possible. If an intra-abdominal testis is detected after puberty, orchidectomy should be performed, as the testis is incapable of spermatogenesis and the risk of malignancy is up to 10 times higher than in a normal testis. If the cord structures enter the internal ring, inguinal exploration is warranted. In boys with bilateral undescended testis in whom neither testis is palpable, chromosomal and endocrine evaluation is needed.

Possible indications for circumcision for patients with phimosis
- Recurrent infection under foreskin
- Appreciable restriction to urine flow

Sites of undescended testis
- Inguinal canal (80%)
- Intra-abdominal (19%)
- Other (1%):
  Suprapubic
  Femoral
  Perineal
  Contralateral scrotum

Main findings on laparascopy to locate an impalpable testis
- Blind ending spermatic vessels above internal inguinal ring but no testis
- Intra-abdominal testis
- Cord structures that enter internal ring

Fertility of an undescended testis becomes compromised after the age of two years

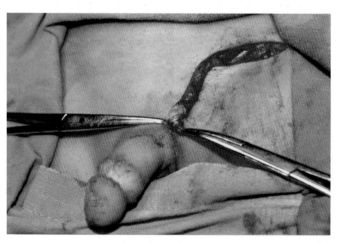

Inguinal exploration of undecended testis

Retractile testis

Retractile testis is common in general practice and is often confused with undescended testis. The key to distinguishing a retractile testis from an undescended testis is to show that the testis can be delivered into the scrotum. A retractile testis will stay in the scrotum after the cremaster muscle has been overstretched, whereas a low undescended testis will immediately pop back to its undescended position after being released. If any doubt exists, the child should be seen in follow up for a repeat examination. If doubt exists as to whether the testis is retractile or undescended, referral for a urological opinion should be arranged.

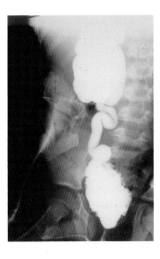

Right sided vesicoureteric junction reflux with gross hydronephrosis

Vesicoureteric junction reflux

Reflux stops spontaneously in a large proportion of patients, although the degree of resolution is inversely proportional to the severity of the reflux. For children with reflux of grades I-II, antibiotic prophylaxis is the recommended initial treatment. In all children with reflux of grades III-V and those with persistent reflux despite a trial of observation on prophylactic antibiotics, surgical correction is recommended. Dysfunctional voiding as a result of bladder instability should be treated with anticholinergic agents.

In the neonatal period, reflux is likely to be the result of anatomical abnormalities; the incidence of reflux is equal in the sexes. In later childhood, the condition predominantly occurs in girls with voiding disturbances. Much evidence shows that reflux should not be considered in isolation and that dysfunctional voiding has a large role in the development of symptoms.

A vicious cycle of symptoms may also exist, because reflux may lead to infection, which itself may lead to bladder instability, dysfunctional voiding, and further reflux. These three elements thus should be considered equally in the treatment of reflux. Reflux alone is now believed not to lead to renal damage—infection also must be present. Many urologists believe that renal damage occurs early in the natural course of the disease, and in many cases it is not progressive.

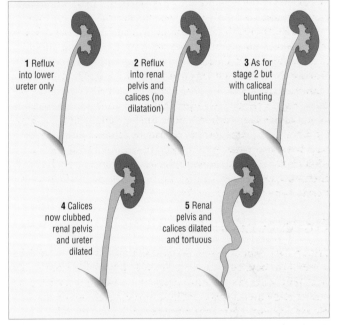

1 Reflux into lower ureter only

2 Reflux into renal pelvis and calices (no dilatation)

3 As for stage 2 but with caliceal blunting

4 Calices now clubbed, renal pelvis and ureter dilated

5 Renal pelvis and calices dilated and tortuous

Grading of vesicoureteric reflux

Recent advances in management of reflux

- Past treatment for reflux centred on ureteric reimplantation
- Recently, endoscopic injection of tetrafluoroethylene polymer (Teflon) into the submucosa of the ureter has been used with some success
- Concern about the risks of migration of particles of tetrafluoroethylene polymer has prevented universal acceptance of the technique
- Other agents, such as bovine crosslinked collagen, autologous chondrocytes, dextranomer plus hyaluronic acid, copolymer and polydimethylsiloxane, have been suggested for injection
- Success rates vary between 65% and 90%

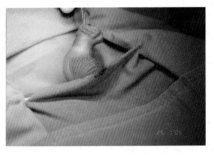

Mid-penile hypospadias

Hypospadias

Hypospadias is a congenital condition that affects three in 1000 male infants and results in underdevelopment of the urethra. The penis may be deviated by chordee, and the urethral opening may be situated anywhere from the perineum to the

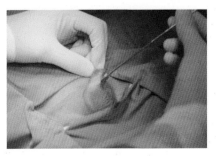

Mid-penile hypospadias— urethral opening calibrated

glans on the ventral surface (in contrast to epispadias in which the opening is on the dorsal surface).

The child should be referred for urological assessment and surgical treatment. The ideal age for surgery is 6–12 months.

Neonatal hydronephrosis

Fetal urinary tract anomalies are common; they occur in 0.2–0.9% of all pregnancies. Hydronephrosis accounts for more than 50% of these anomalies. Antenatal hydronephrosis may be caused by ureteropelvic junction obstruction, ureterovesical junction obstruction, multicystic kidney, primary obstructive megaureter, vesicoureteral reflux, or posterior urethral valves.

In cases of mild unilateral hydronephrosis (<15 mm in diameter) with normal appearing renal parenchyma, further prenatal follow up is seldom useful, and surgery is unnecessary. A postnatal check is important to confirm the hydronephrosis has resolved.

In cases of moderate unilateral hydronephrosis (15–19 mm), ultrasound and a micturating cystogram should be performed at two months and subsequently at intervals of six months. Surgery also is unlikely to be needed in these cases.

In cases of severe unilateral hydronephrosis (>20 mm), ultrasound, a micturating cystogram, and an isotopic renal scan should be performed at one month. Severe unilateral hydronephrosis is most likely eventually to need surgery.

In neonates with severe bilateral hydronephrosis, ultrasound and a micturating cystogram should be performed within one week. Early surgery is often indicated.

Obstruction of pelviureteric junction

The essential defect seems to be an aperistaltic segment of ureter, from which the normal musculature is congenitally absent. The role of "aberrant" vessels in causing obstruction recently has been questioned. These vessels are usually normal variants, often pass behind the ureter, and are not generally thought to cause obstruction.

It is usually diagnosed by intravenous urography, which shows delay in appearance of contrast on the affected side and dilated renal pelvis and calices. The ureter, when seen, is usually not dilated. Differential renal function and confirmation of obstruction should be obtained with isotope renography.

Surgery is indicated for obstructive symptoms, stone formation, recurrent urinary infection, or progressive renal impairment. Pyeloplasty is the treatment of choice, but if the affected kidney possesses <10% of total renal function, nephrectomy should be performed. Minimally invasive alternative techniques include antegrade endopyelotomy and laparoscopic pyeloplasty. Laparoscopic pyeloplasty is becoming the treatment of choice, and open procedures usually are reserved for patients in whom laparoscopic surgery is contraindicated.

Common paediatric tumours

Wilms' tumour

Wilms' tumour (nephroblastoma) is the most common primary malignant renal tumour of childhood. It typically affects young children (median age 3.5 years), with more than 80% of the patients being identified before the age of five years. The most common presentation of Wilms' tumour is an abdominal mass, although haematuria is the presenting feature in up to 15% of cases. Wilms' tumour is usually diagnosed with ultrasound, computed tomography, or magnetic resonance imaging.

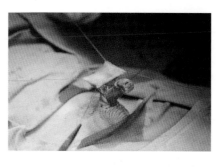

Hypospadias surgery—transverse preputial island flap

The use of routine ultrasound examination in pregnancy has identified a number of fetuses with hydronephrosis. Postnatal evaluation and management depends on the severity and laterality of hydronephrosis

Presentation of pelviureteric obstruction

- Obstruction of the pelviureteric junction may occur at any time (before birth, in childhood, or in adulthood)
- Infants typically present with an abdominal mass
- Older children may have abdominal pain
- The condition often presents with haematuria after fairly minor abdominal trauma

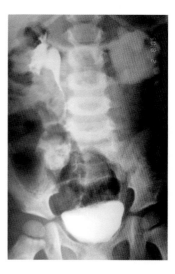

Congenital obstruction of left pelvi-ureteric junction

Wilms' tumour

- About 15% of children with Wilms' tumour have congenital abnormalities, including musculoskeletal and other genitourinary anomalies (4.4%)
- Bilateral disease is seen in 5–7% of children with Wilms' tumour

Wilms' tumour is treated by radical nephrectomy; chemotherapy is usually given after surgery, with the exact protocol depending on the stage of the disease. Radiotherapy is needed only if residual tumour has been left behind at surgery and for patients with lymphatic and pulmonary metastases. Neoadjuvant chemotherapy is beneficial for patients with bilateral involvement.

Renal cell carcinoma

This tumour is rare in children and is not usually diagnosed until confirmed by histological examination of a presumed Wilms' tumour. Some tumours are chemosensitive, and radiotherapy may be needed for microscopic residual disease, but radical nephrectomy remains the mainstay of treatment.

Rhabdomyosarcoma

This sarcoma commonly presents with lower urinary tract symptoms, particularly haematuria or urinary retention. Tumours of the vagina may cause a foul vaginal discharge, and pelvic tumours may cause a large mass.

Rhabdomyosarcoma is treated effectively with chemotherapy. The role of radical surgery is diminishing and currently is reserved for children who fail to respond to chemotherapy or develop a pelvic relapse.

References

- Rickwood AMK. Medical indications for circumcision. *BJU Int* 1999;83:45–51.
- Elder JS. Abnormalities of the genitalia in boys and their surgical management. In: Walsh PC, Retik AB, Vaughn ED, Wein AJ, eds. *Campbell's urology*. Philadelphia, PA: Saunders, 2002:2334–52.
- Kolon TF, Patel RP, Huff DS. Cryptoorchidism: diagnosis, treatment and long-term prognosis. *Urol Clin N Am* 2004;31:469–80.
- Austin JC, Cooper CS. Vesicoureteral reflux: surgical approaches. *Urol Clin N Am* 2004;31:543–57.

12 Genitourinary trauma

Asif Muneer

Trauma is defined as a morbid condition of the body produced by external violence. The genitourinary structures most commonly involved are the kidneys and testicles.

Renal trauma

Renal trauma is the most common genitourinary injury and accounts for 1–5% of all trauma. The incidence of renal trauma is higher in men than women. The availability of high resolution imaging modalities and staging of trauma has led to a reduction in the need for surgical intervention and thus increased renal preservation.

Mechanism of injury

The mechanism of injury may be blunt trauma or penetrating injuries. Blunt trauma most often occurs as a result of road traffic accidents. The remaining cases are attributed to assaults, falls, and contact sports.

Penetrating renal injuries occur as a result of gunshot and stab wounds. The highest rates are within urban areas as a result of gang violence and street crime. These account for severe and unpredictable injuries. The passage of a bullet through the abdomen can result in multiple organ injuries, with significant renal parenchymal destruction. Gunshot wounds are classified as high velocity and low velocity. Low velocity gunshot wounds produce a blast effect that results in damage to the tissues. High velocity gunshot wounds cause more associated injuries.

Classification

Several classification systems have been used over the years according to the morphological findings and clinical course. The most widely accepted classification system is that of the American Association for the Surgery of Trauma, which classifies renal injuries on a scale of 1–5.

Diagnosis

All patients with trauma need an initial assessment that includes securing the airway, control of external bleeding, and cardiovascular resuscitation. This should follow the criteria of the advanced trauma and life support system.

The history from a conscious patient or witness (in the case of a severely injured patient) may indicate a major renal injury. Direct blows to the flank or an event that involved rapid deceleration lead to a high index of suspicion. The type and size of the weapon and the velocity of the gunshot are valuable points of information if available. If the patient is conscious, any pre-existing renal pathology or renal dysfunction should be documented, as they may complicate even minor renal injuries.

Physical examination involves assessment of haemodynamic stability. The presence of shock may be determined with a simplified classification that involves blood loss, heart rate, blood pressure, pulse pressure, respiratory rate, and mental state. Other signs that indicate an underlying renal injury include fractured ribs, flank ecchymoses or abrasions, abdominal tenderness, or distension associated with flank pain.

Urinalysis is a basic test in the evaluation of patients with trauma. Microscopic haematuria in the trauma setting is defined as more than five red blood cells per high powered field;

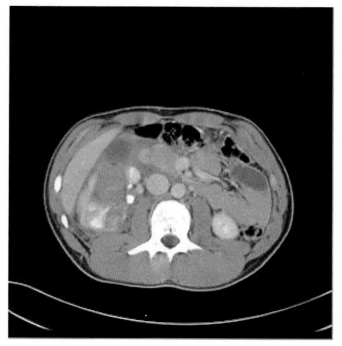

Computed tomography scan showing significant injury after blunt renal trauma

Classification of renal injuries

Grade	Description of injury
1	Contusion or non-expanding subcapsular haematoma No laceration
2	Non-expanding perirenal haematoma Cortical laceration <1 cm
3	Cortical laceration >1 cm
4	Laceration through corticomedullary junction into collecting system or Segmental artery or vein injury with contained haematoma
5	Shattered kidney or renal pedicle injury or avulsion

Simplified classification of haemorrhagic shock

Feature	Class			
	1	2	3	4
Blood loss (%)	<15	15–30	30–40	>40
Heart rate (beats/minute)	<100	>100	>120	>140
Blood pressure (mm Hg)	Normal	Normal	Decreased	Decreased
Pulse pressure	Normal or increased	Decreased	Decreased	Decreased
Respiratory rate (breaths/minute)	14–20	20–30	30–40	>35
Mental state	Slightly anxious	Mildly anxious	Anxious, confused	Confused, lethargic

Adapted from www.tarn.ac.uk/research/Abstracts/guly1.pdf

Major renal injuries may occur without haematuria

macroscopic haematuria is blood readily visible in a urine specimen. The degree of haematuria, however, does not always correlate with the magnitude of the renal trauma.

Imaging

Not all injuries need imaging for further assessment. Large studies have concluded that patients with blunt trauma and microscopic haematuria without shock are unlikely to have a significant renal injury and thus do not need imaging. The preferred imaging method for stable patients with renal trauma is computed tomography.

Management

Most blunt injuries are managed conservatively. Life threatening haemodynamic instability or grade 5 injuries, however, are an absolute indication for surgical exploration. The overall exploration rate after blunt trauma is <10%. Most explorations ultimately lead to a nephrectomy, depending on the nature and severity of the injury. Reconstruction, in the form of renorraphy, can be performed in some cases at surgery. The presence of a normal functioning kidney on the contralateral side must be established; this is usually achieved with a one shot intravenous pyelogram before surgery.

Laparotomy is usually needed to explore intraperitoneal non-renal injuries—such as occur after penetrating trauma to the bowel, liver, or spleen. Although these organs require repair or resection, the simultaneous presence of a non-expanding retroperitoneal haematoma is best managed by leaving it undisturbed.

Follow up involves serial measurements of blood pressure and renal function. The use of radiological imaging during follow up depends on whether reconstruction or conservative management is used.

Paediatric renal trauma

The kidneys lie lower in children than in adults and are protected less well by the abdominal muscles and lower ribs. Children therefore are more susceptible to blunt renal trauma.

A full history and examination are essential to evaluate the mechanism of injury and any pre-existing renal disease. Unlike in adults, the absence of hypotension is an unreliable sign in children, as significant loss of blood still can be associated with a relatively stable blood pressure.

Ultrasound can be used as an imaging method in children who are stable, but computed tomography is mandatory to accurately stage the injury.

Testicular injuries

Testicular injuries can be classified as blunt and penetrating injuries. Blunt traumas that arise from kicks or straddle injuries compress the testis against the lower border of the pubic bone and can result in minor contusion or complete rupture of the tunica albuginea. Significant testicular injuries present with a swollen tender scrotum. Ultrasound assessment can be used to differentiate between testicular contusion or rupture, but the accuracy is limited.

Management

Testicular trauma in the absence of significant scrotal swelling can be managed conservatively. Early scrotal exploration is needed in cases of testicular rupture, and devitalised tissue is removed, with repair of the tunica albuginea. Non-viable testicles are removed by orchidectomy.

Penetrating trauma to the testicle may be secondary to a gunshot wound or stabbing. Debridement of non-viable tissue is undertaken, with an attempt to preserve as much testicular

Indications for further radiological imaging in patients with blunt renal trauma

Haematuria on urinalysis	Haemodynamic status	Imaging needed
Microscopic	No shock	No imaging
Macroscopic	No shock	Computed tomography
Macroscopic	Shock	Computed tomography if stable or intravenous urogram on table if unstable

In patients with renal trauma, computed tomography is a more sensitive and specific method than other imaging methods, such as intravenous pyelography, ultrasound, and angiography

Non-operative management of patients with renal trauma involves bed rest and adequate hydration; <5% of patients fail conservative management

Complications of renal trauma

Early complications	Late complications
• Bleeding	• Hydronephrosis
• Infection	• Calculus formation
• Abscess formation	• Chronic pyelonephritis
• Urinary fistula	• Hypertension (Page kidney)
• Hypertension	• Arteriovenous fistula
• Urinoma	• Pseudoaneurysm

Testicular injuries are common during aggressive sports and motor vehicle crashes because of the vulnerable position of the male genitalia

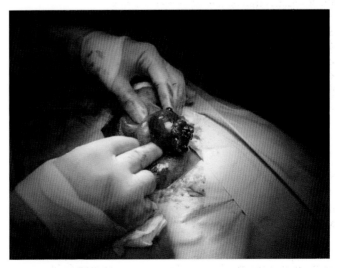

Testicular rupture

tissue as possible. When the testicle cannot be conserved, orchidectomy is performed. Broad spectrum antibiotics are needed, and the tetanus status of the patient must be checked.

Penile fracture

Extreme angulation of the erect penis during sexual intercourse accounts for most penile fractures. The classic history is diagnostic, and the tear in the tunica sometimes can be palpated. In uncertain cases, magnetic resonance imaging of the penis will differentiate between a complete tunical tear and intracavernosal haematoma. A tunical tear needs immediate exploration of the penis to evacuate the haematoma and repair the injury.

> **Early repair of penile fracture maintains erectile function and prevents late onset penile curvature**

Urethral injuries

In men, the urethra is divided into posterior and anterior segments by the urogenital diaphragm. Posterior urethral injuries most commonly occur as a result of pelvic fractures sustained in road traffic accidents, falls from a height, and crush injuries. The injury can range from a stretch or contusion injury to complete disruption of the posterior urethra. Anterior urethral injuries are rarely associated with pelvic fractures but can occur after road traffic accidents, falls, or straddle type injuries that involve a blunt blow to the perineum. Iatrogenic injury to the urethra secondary to endoscopic trauma and instrumentation is the most common cause of urethral stricture.

Diagnosis

Presence of blood at the urethral meatus should lead to a high index of suspicion of an underlying urethral injury. Retrograde urethrography should be performed before catheterisation of the urethra is tried. If a urethral injury is diagnosed by retrograde urethrography, a suprapubic catheter is inserted. Initial diagnosis and management should focus on avoiding further injury.

Management

Penetrating injuries to the anterior urethra can be repaired by primary anastomosis over a urethral catheter. Anterior urethral injuries associated with stricture formation can be managed with endoscopy for short strictures or urethroplasty for longer strictures. Management of posterior urethral injuries is more complex and must take into account associated injuries. If the patient is stable and can tolerate the lithotomy position, delayed primary end to end urethroplasty can be done within two weeks. Alternatives are realignment, which can be performed as an open or endoscopic procedure, or delayed urethroplasty.

Bladder injuries

Iatrogenic trauma and direct blunt trauma account for most cases of bladder rupture. As the bladder has intraperitoneal and extraperitoneal components, the degree of bladder distension at the time of injury determines whether an intraperitoneal or extraperitoneal leak is likely. The site of bladder rupture governs the subsequent management.

Classic presentation of penile fracture
- Severe pain
- Rapid detumescence
- Penile swelling as a result of rupture of the tunica albuginea that covers the corpora cavernosa.

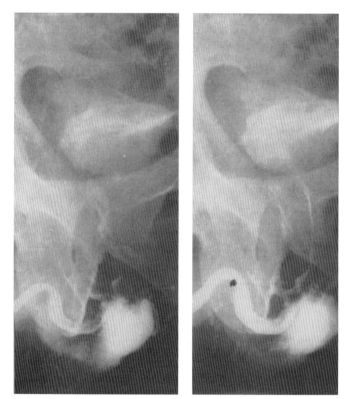

Rapid detumescence and penile swelling accompany a penile fracture

> **Posterior urethra comprises membranous and prostatic urethra; anterior urethra consists of bulbar and penile urethra**

> **Patients who need realignment and delayed urethroplasty for urethral injuries are usually referred to a specialist centre**

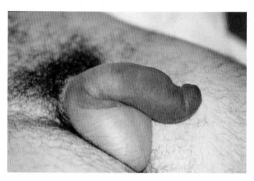

Urethrogram showing urethral rupture

Diagnosis

Gross haematuria occurs in up to 82% of patients, along with lower abdominal tenderness. Retrograde cystography will confirm if the rupture is intraperitoneal or extraperitoneal.

Management

Blunt extraperitoneal rupture can be managed safely by catheter drainage, ensuring that the catheter does not get blocked by clots. Most ruptures heal within 10 days. Intraperitoneal rupture can be complicated by peritonitis as a result of a urinary leak and must always undergo surgical exploration with repair of the bladder laceration.

Further reading

Weiss RM, George NJR, O'Reilly PH. *Comprehensive urology*. St Louis, MO: Mosby, 2000.

Index

α-agonists 16
α-blockers 7, 9
adhesins, bacterial 22
alfuzosin 7
alpha fetoprotein 35, 36
anal sphincter examination 3
androgen deficiency 21
andrology x
andropause 21
antiandrogens 28
antibiotics 2, 23, 24, 46
antimuscarinic drugs 12
antisperm antibody testing 18–19
aromatic amines 29
arterial steal syndrome 16
assisted reproductive techniques 19

bacterial cell adhesion 22
bacterial pathogens 22
bacteriuria screening 24
balloon dilatation of prostatic fossa 9
BCG (bacille Calmette–Guérin),
    intravesical 31, 32
benign prostatic hyperplasia 6, 14
bicalutamide 28
biofeedback training 11
bisphosphonates 28
bladder
    augmentation 12
    bacteria 22
    biopsy 30, 31
    capacity 11
    compliance 11
    detrusor overactivity 10, 12
    detrusor pressure 11
    distended 14
    drainage 23
    emptying 7
    injuries 46–7
    innervation 3
    myomectomy 12
    rupture 46–7
    ultrasound examination 4
bladder cancer ix, 29–33
    aetiology 29
    carcinoma in situ 31–2
    diagnosis 30
    investigations 29–30
    metastases 30, 32
    muscle invasive 32
    palliative care 33
    signs/symptoms 29
    staging 30
    superficial 30–2
    treatment 30–3
    UTI differential diagnosis 23
bladder neck
    dysfunction/dyssynergia 6, 9
    incision 9
    obstruction 6
bladder outflow obstruction 6–9
    examination 6

investigations 6–7
surgical intervention 7–9
symptoms 1, 6
treatment 7–9
bone scans, isotope 5, 26
brachytherapy 27
bulbocavernosal reflex loss 16

calcium oxalate 39
carcinogenesis, two hit hypothesis 34
carcinogens, industrial 29
catheterisation
    bladder trauma 47
    suprapubic 46
    urethral 14, 17, 46
chemotherapy
    adjuvant 32
    neoadjuvant 32, 43
    renal cancer 35, 43
    rhabdomyosarcoma 43
    testicular cancer 36
    Wilms' tumour 43
children x, 40–3
    renal trauma 45
    testicular torsion 15
    tumours 42–3
choriocarcinoma 35, 36
chromosomal abnormalities,
    subfertility 18
cigarette smoking 29
circumcision 16, 40
clam cystoplasty 12
computed tomography (CT) 5
    prostate cancer staging 26
    testicular cancer 36
congenital anomalies ix, 42
creatinine, serum levels 4
cremasteric reflex 3
crush injuries 46
cryotherapy
    prostate 27
    renal cancer 35
cyproterone acetate 28
cystectomy 33
    radical 31, 32
cystitis 23
cystography, retrograde 47
cystoplasty, clam 12
cystoprostatectomy 32
cystoscopy 13, 30

detrusor instability management 12
detrusor overactivity 10, 12
detrusor pressure 11
diet, stone disease 39
dimercaptosuccinic acid (DMSA) 5
dipstick testing 2, 3, 24
doxazosin 7
dutasteride 7
dysuria 1

EDTA clearance 5

Index

ejaculation
  dysfunction 18
  failure 2
  premature 2
  retrograde 2, 7, 9, 18, 19
emergencies, urological 14–17
endometriosis 12
endopyelotomy, antegrade 42
endoscopy, urethral strictures 46
epididymis
  examination 3, 24
  ultrasound examination 4
epididymitis 15
epididymo-orchitis 24
erectile dysfunction x, 2, 18
  subfertility 19–20
Escherichia coli 22
extracorporeal shockwave
    lithotripsy 15, 38
extraurethral incontinence 10, 11

fertility problems x, 18–19, 40
fever 2
finasteride 7
foreskin 16, 40

genitalia, external 2–3
genitourinary tract examination 2–3
glans penis 16
glomerular filtration rate measurement 5
gunshot injuries 44, 45

haematuria 23
  bladder cancer 29
  bladder trauma 47
  macroscopic 45
  microscopic 15, 29, 44, 45
  rhabdomyosarcoma 43
  Wilms' tumour 42
haemodynamic stability 44
healthcare professionals xi
hormone therapy, prostate cancer 27
human chorionic gonadotrophin
    (hCG) 35–6
hydatid of Morgagni 15
hydronephrosis 2, 41
  neonatal 42
hypercalciuria 39
hypospadias 19, 41–2
hysterectomy 32
  vesicovaginal fistula risk 12

ileal conduit 32
immunotherapy, renal cancer 35
incontinence nurse practitioners xi, 11
infertility x, 18–19
innovations xi
interferon α 35
interleukin 2 (IL-2) 35
International prostate symptom score
    (IPSS) 6
intracavernosal haematoma 46
intracavernosal pharmacotherapy 20
intracytoplasmic sperm injection 19
investigations 3–4
in-vitro fertilisation (IVF) 19
irritative symptoms 1

kidney
  infections 2, 15, 17, 24
  obstruction 17, 24
  percutaneous drainage 24

surgical reconstruction 45
trauma 44–5
ultrasound examination 4
see also renal *entries*

lactate dehydrogenase 36
laparoscopic surgery x, xi
  prostate cancer 28
  pyeloplasty 42
laparoscopy
  pyeloplasty 42
  undescended testis 40
laparotomy, intraperitoneal injuries 45
laser therapy, bladder obstruction 8
lithotripsy ix, 15, 38
Lue procedure 20
luteinizing hormone-releasing hormone agonists 28

magnetic resonance imaging (MRI) 5
  prostate cancer staging 26
male, ageing 21
mercaptoacetylglycine (MAG3) 5
metastases
  bladder cancer 30, 32
  immunotherapy 35
  isotope bone scans 26
  prostate cancer 16, 28
  radiotherapy 35
  spinal cord compression 16, 17
  testicular cancer 36
  Wilms' tumour 43
microwave hyperthermia 8
micturating cystogram 42
micturition
  frequency 1–2
  symptoms 1
mitomycin C 31
myomectomy, bladder 12

needle ablation, transurethral of prostate 8
nephrectomy
  pelviureteric junction obstruction 42
  renal cancer 35, 43
  renal trauma 45
  Wilms' tumour 43
nephrolithotomy, percutaneous 38
nephrostomy, percutaneous 2, 15
  bladder cancer 33
nephrostomy drainage 2, 24
Nesbitt operation 20
nocturnal enuresis 17
nuclear medicine 5
nurse practitioners, specialist xi, 11

obstructive symptoms 1
oligospermia 18
oncology ix
orchidectomy
  emergency 16
  radical 36
  testicular trauma 46
orchidopexy 40
overflow incontinence 10, 11

p53 mutation 34
pad testing 10
paediatric disorders x, 40–3
  renal trauma 45
  tumours 42–3
palliative care
  bladder cancer 33
  prostate cancer 28

paradoxical incontinence 10
paraphimosis 16
pelvic clearance, anterior 32
pelvic floor training 11, 12
pelvic fractures 46
pelvic node dissection 32
pelviureteric junction obstruction 42
penile prostheses 20
penile ring block 16
penis
    arteriovenous shunt 16
    aspiration of corpora 16
    curvature 20
    examination 3
    fracture 46
Peyronie's disease 3, 20
phenylephrine 16
phimosis 40
phosphodiesterase inhibitors 19–20
photo selective vaporization of prostate
        with green light laser 8
positron emission tomography (PET) 5
pregnancy, urinary tract infection 24
prepuce, adhesions 40
priapism 15–16, 17
prostaglandin E$_1$, intracavernosal injection 20
prostate
    biopsy 26, 27
    cryotherapy 27
    examination 3, 24
    medical therapy of symptoms 7
    stenting 8–9
    surgical intervention 7–9
    ultrasound examination 4
    volume reduction 7
    see also benign prostatic hyperplasia
prostate cancer ix, 25–8
    active surveillance 26–7
    epidemiology 25
    investigation 25–6
    laparoscopic surgery 28
    localised 26–7
    locally advanced 27
    management 26
    metastases 16, 28
    palliative care 28
    robotic surgery 28
    screening 26
    staging 26
    symptoms/signs 25
    urine retention 14
prostatectomy
    open 9
    radical 27, 28
prostate-specific antigen (PSA) 6–7, 25
prostatic fossa, balloon dilatation 9
prostatitis 24
proteomics 28
pyelography, intravenous 30
pyelonephritis 15, 24
pyeloplasty 42

radiofrequency ablation, renal cancer 35
radiology 5
    renal cell carcinoma 34
radiotherapy
    external beam 27
    pain relief 28
    pelvic 12
    renal cancer metastases 35
    renal cell carcinoma 43
    Wilms' tumour 43

reconstruction procedures ix–x
rectal examination 3, 24
5α-reductase inhibitors 7
renal calculi/stones 15, 37
    investigations 37
    staghorn 38
    treatment 38, 39
renal cancer/renal cell carcinoma 34–5
    children 43
    staging 34
    treatment 35
renal colic 2, 14–15, 17
renal function 4
renal transplantation x
renal trauma 44–5
renal ultrasound 24
renography, dynamic isotope/static 5
renorrhaphy 45
renoscopy, retrograde 38
retroperitoneal haematoma 45
retroperitoneal lymph node dissection 36
rhabdomyosarcoma 43
road traffic accidents 44, 46
robotic surgery, prostate cancer 28

salpingo-oophorectomy 32
saw palmetto 7
scrotum
    examination 2–3
    trauma 45
    ultrasound examination 4
self-catheterisation, intermittent 12
semen analysis 18
seminoma 35, 36
sexual dysfunction 2
shared care xi
shock 44
sperm banks 36
sperm extraction 19
spinal cord compression 16, 28
stabbings 45
Staphylococcus saprophyticus 22
stents
    prostate 8–9
    ureteric 24
stone disease ix, 2, 37–9
    investigations 37
    metabolic screening 39
    presentation 37
    recurrence 39
    renal colic 15
    stone composition 39
    treatment 38–9
    ureteric 4
strangury 1, 2, 37
stress incontinence 10, 11
    surgical management 12
strontium 28
subfertility x, 18–19
    undescended testis 40
support groups 11
surgery x
symptoms 1–2

tamsulosin 7
terbutaline 16
testes
    examination 3, 24
    intra-abdominal 40
    retractile 41
    rupture 45
    trauma 45–6

Index

testes (*contd.*)
  ultrasound examination 4
  undescended 40
testicular cancer 15, 35–6
  germ cell 35
  markers 35–6
  metastases 36
  undescended testis 40
testicular torsion 3, 15, 17
testosterone therapy 21
tetrafluoroethylene polymer ureteral injection 41
three swab test 13
TNM classification 26
training x, xi
transurethral incision of the prostate 8
transurethral microwave therapy 8
transurethral needle ablation of the prostate 8
transurethral resection of the prostate 8, 9
trauma 44–7
trigonitis 23
tunical tear 46

ultrasound 4
  bladder cancer 30
  children 45
  high intensity focused 8, 27
  hydronephrosis 42
  prostate 26
  renal 24, 34, 42
  renal cell carcinoma 34
ureter
  dilatation 4
  obstruction 37
  submucosal tetrafluoroethylene
    polymer injection 41
  ultrasound examination 4
ureteric calculi/stones 4, 15, 37
  investigations 37
  treatment 38–9
ureteric colic 2
ureteric stents 24
ureterography, retrograde 13
ureterolithotomy, endoscopic 38
ureteroscopy 15
urethra
  catheterisation 14, 17, 46
  injuries 46
  ruptured 17
  strictures 6, 9, 14, 46
  underdevelopment 41
urethral meatus 3
  blood 46
  tight 23
urethral sphincter, artificial 12
urethrography, retrograde 46
urethroplasty, urethral strictures 46
urge incontinence 10, 12

urgency 1
urinalysis 10
urinary diversion 32, 33
urinary incontinence 2, 10–13
  assessment 10–11
  examination 10
  postoperative 27
  reconstruction procedures ix–x
  surgical management 12
  treatment 11–12
urinary stream 1
urinary tract, upper
  infection 15, 24
  obstruction 24
urinary tract infection 22–4
  differential diagnosis 23
  lower 2
  management 22–4
  men 24
  pregnancy 24
  recurrent 23
  stone disease 39
  upper 15, 24
  women 22–4
urine
  biochemistry 4
  culture 3
  cytology 3–4
  dipstick testing 2, 3, 22
  flow rate 7
  leakage 2, 10
  midstream sample 22, 23
  residual volume 7
  retention 7, 14, 27
    rhabdomyosarcoma 43
  voiding dysfunction 41
urodynamic disorders ix, x
urodynamic investigations 5, 11
uroflowmetry 10
urography, intravenous 5, 13
urological complaints 1
urological evaluation 1–5
urological practice x
urology nurse practitioners xi, 11

vacuum devices 20
vaginectomy 32
varicocelectomy 18–19
vesical pressure 11
vesicoureteric junction reflux 41
vesicovaginal fistula 10, 12–13
videourodynamics 11
Von Hippel-Lindau disease 34

Wilms' tumour 42–3

zoledronic acid 28